YOU ARE
BEAUTIFUL

Ken Paves

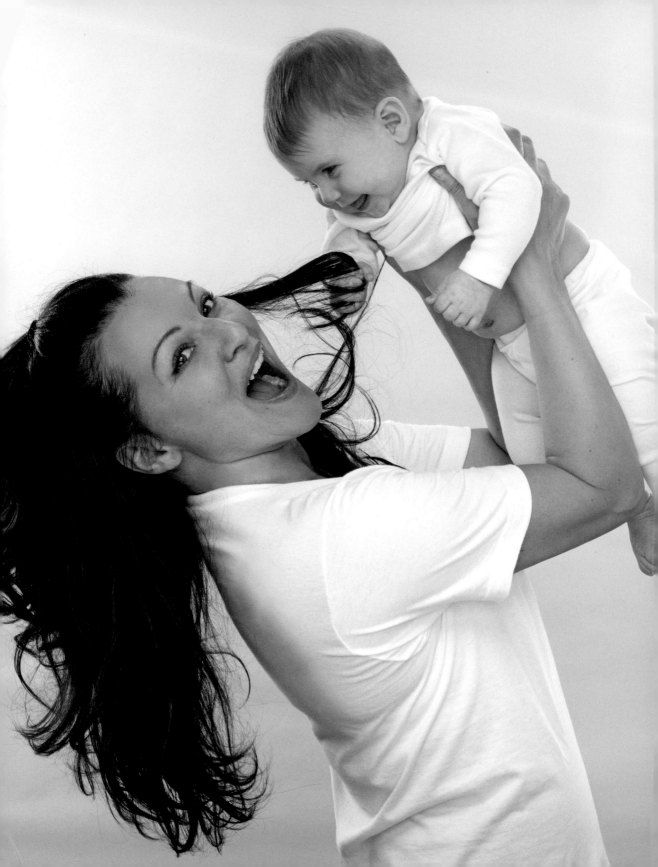

YOU ARE
BEAUTIFUL

A BEAUTY GUIDE FOR *REAL WOMEN*

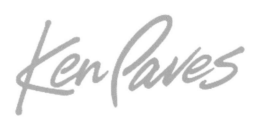

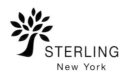

STERLING
New York

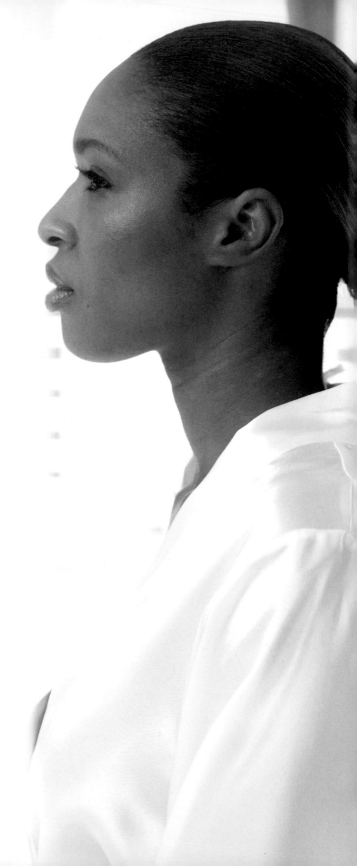

STERLING
New York

An Imprint of Sterling Publishing
387 Park Avenue South
New York, NY 10016

A Buoy Point Media Production
Interior Design: Fabia Wargin

Photography Credits
15: © Brian Hirsch; 37: © Disney;
Throughout: "real women" studio
photography © Richard Mclaren

Every effort has been made to credit photographers
whose work appears in this book. In the event we
inadvertently omitted credit lines, we encourage
photographers to contact us in order to be credited
for their work in future reprints of this book.

ISBN 978-1-4027-9708-8

Distributed in Canada by Sterling Publishing
c/o Canadian Manda Group
165 Dufferin Street
Toronto, Ontario, Canada M6K 3H6
Distributed in the United Kingdom by
GMC Distribution Services
Castle Place, 166 High Street
Lewes, East Sussex, England BN7 1XU
Distributed in Australia by
Capricorn Link (Australia) Pty. Ltd.
P.O. Box 704, Windsor, NSW 2756, Australia

For information about custom editions, special sales,
and premium and corporate purchases, please contact
Sterling Special Sales at 800-805-5489 or
specialsales@sterlingpublishing.com.

Manufactured in China

2 4 6 8 10 9 7 5 3 1

www.sterlingpublishing.com

CONTENTS

*I dedicate this book to
one of the most beautiful and loving women
I have ever known, my grandmother,*

LOUISE FELARCA
(1918-2012).

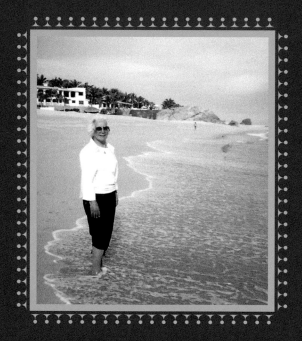

My grandfather passed away at an early age, and my grandmother was left to
raise eight children, alone, in the 1950s. She worked full-time as a nurse,
raised her children, and was the best grandmother ever!
She inspired me beyond measure.
She worked tirelessly and loved endlessly.
She was BEAUTIFUL!
I miss you, Gram mama—You are my beautiful butterfly!

FOREWORD

KENNEY, KENNEY, KENNEY

I started working with Kenney nearly nine years ago. I watched him from afar, admiring his work, wishing to work with him one day. Little did I know he was trying to do the same! Finally I got the chance to meet him one night at a movie premiere. He was standing with Eva Mendez and I walked over and said, "Hi, I'm Eva, and I am a big fan of your work, and I would love to work with you one day." He stared at me with a blank face and then nodded his head. He didn't say anything; no words came out of his mouth—he just smiled, nodded, and then walked away. I was heartbroken! I thought, "Oh no! He doesn't like me and doesn't want to work with me!" Later I found out he was so nervous to meet me that he couldn't speak!

Knowing Kenney now, it all makes sense. Despite being a hair genius, a celebrity hairstylist, a hair guru to the stars, and a bold and successful entrepreneur, he really is shy! In fact, he's so shy that anywhere we go he hangs onto my arm and won't let go, or he cowers in the corners of rooms until he finds someone he knows to talk to. I've always found this a paradox, since Kenney is the most giving, generous, funny, charismatic person I know. Where did this insecurity come from? Where does this shyness live in that beautiful brain of his? I realized it comes from a place in his personality called humility. His humbleness is beautiful to watch and wonderful to be around. I always tell Kenney he could be the worst hairdresser in the world and I would still hire him, because I love being bathed in the light that surrounds him; I love being in the presence of endless talent and creativity; and I love being around a spirit that lifts everyone around him.

I look forward to every shoot we do, sitting in the chair and being a muse for the day. I get to sit back for a short time and let him work the magic that comes out of his mind, into his hands, and onto my hair. I always know that no matter what we are working on—a commercial, a magazine shoot, or the red carpet—I will never have a bad hair day.

I am so happy that Kenney is writing this book, a memoir of his life told through the story of hair. He strives to lift women up and empower them with self-confidence and self-esteem. His secrets should be shared with the world and now they are! His love and appreciation for women of every color and every background shines through his work. Changing our hair allows us to evoke sex appeal, confidence, charisma, poise, self-assurance, validation, sureness, and charm. And I will be forever grateful to him for allowing me to be part of his journey, professionally and personally. I am honored to work with him and humbled to call him my friend and my brother.

—Eva Longoria

INTRODUCTION

Hi, my name is Ken Paves. I want you to help me change the way we define beauty today. Each of you, individually and uniquely, defines true beauty.

As a hairstylist for nearly two decades, I have had the honor and pleasure of working with—and learning so much about beauty from—hundreds of women: stay-at-home moms, single moms, and professional women.

Doing makeovers on women all over the world on *The Oprah Winfrey Show*, *The X Factor*, *The Biggest Loser*, *The Doctors*, *America's Next Top Model*, and in *O! The Oprah Magazine*, among other media outlets, has been perhaps one of the most satisfying parts of my career. All the women I've made over were already beautiful. I had the honor of simply enhancing what they already had. Seeing these wonderful women realize just how gorgeous they were—for the first time, in some cases—and how happy they were (thank goodness!) with the outcome is why I love what I do.

Working with women of all ages, ethnicities, shapes, and sizes for many, many years has allowed me to appreciate all kinds of beauty. Every woman I've ever met has inspired me to see that beauty has no definition. To me, all women are beautiful. That is why I'm writing this book.

I am grateful for the success that I have found in the beauty industry, but along the way I've seen firsthand how the industry's grandiose standards have become impossible for most "real" women to attain. This is hurtful to women everywhere and, sadly, it has made many women think less of themselves.

If you've ever felt this way, then you're in good company. So many of the hundreds of women I've met and worked with over the years have told me they're tired of having someone tell them what they should look like.

I completely understand women's concerns about their looks because I've been there myself. I'm no Brad Pitt. I think I look more like Ellen DeGeneres. I'm also a skinny fat person, skinny but a little flabby. And I'm only five foot eight—or five foot ten if I slip a little something in my shoe. There have been many times in my life when I haven't felt great about myself or who I am. When I was growing up, I didn't feel like I looked like everyone else, and sometimes other kids said hurtful things to me about my appearance.

When I was becoming a hairstylist, I was told not only that I didn't "look like one," but also that, because I came from the "wrong side of town," it would be hard for me to get a job. These comments really hurt, but I used them to become a stronger person. I always like to focus on the positive. And that's what I would like you to do, too. To be honest, today, at forty-one years old, I am very happy with who I am and what I look like. I love that I don't look like anyone else but me. (Well, except my mom!)

I feel that because of the success I've achieved in the beauty industry, I'm obligated to help it evolve. I want to right the wrongs of the industry in which I have become successful and help women everywhere to embrace and own their beauty. After all, it is not necessarily the industry that has made me successful. In fact, it has been all of you—all of the women who have ever appreciated my work—who have made me successful. I owe it to you to do what is right.

This book is about improving the way you feel about yourself. It's about being your own best friend, loving what you see in the mirror, and accepting how beautiful you are on the inside as well as on the outside. It's about discovering and celebrating the inner radiance that tells the world how special and unique you are.

You don't ever have to beat yourself up over your looks. You don't have to compare yourself to an airbrushed, nipped and tucked, super-styled supermodel or celebrity (who doesn't even look like that in real life) or to some absurd, impossible standard of beauty that doesn't really exist. You don't have to meet anyone's standards except your own. When you've finished reading this book, I would love for you to put it down and say, "Damn it, I am beautiful. I'm finished with the struggle. I'm finished with the fight. I am me. If people don't love me as I am, then that's their issue. I'm going to have a wonderful life, loving who I am right now."

Coming to terms with your own beauty starts with self-acceptance. Women can be very hard on themselves for no reason. Do you have a couple of extra pounds around your middle? So what? You still look great! Do you think your hair looks too fine and flat? Learn to work with it, instead of against it.

So forget about what you think you're supposed to look like and embrace what you *do* look like. Happy the way you are already? Fantastic! But if there are some things you want to change for yourself— not for your husband, your significant other, your mother, your kids, your friends, or the catty girls at work—but for *you*—I'm going to share the tips I give to my clients and the women I make over, to help bring out the best in you.

The key, of course, is confidence—a woman's most powerful acces-sory. That confidence tells the world just how beautiful you truly are, but first you have to believe it yourself.

As for that inner radiance I was talking about? I'll let you in on a little secret. You already have that inside of you. Maybe you don't think it's there, but it is. My goal is to help you find that inner glow. And when you do? I want you to show it to the world.

My hope is that this is the kind of book you will refer to again and again, not just for beauty and hair tips, but for inspiration to help you get through a trying moment or a tough day. My goal is to help you feel better about yourself so those good feelings will carry over to all aspects of your life.

I look forward to accompanying you on this life-changing journey. It may take a little work, time, and self-exploration on your part, but the results will all be worth it. And we will definitely have fun along the way.

We are going to start a revolution with *You Are Beautiful*. We will band together and show the world just how many beautiful women are out there. Together, we can make a difference. So forget about what you think you should look like. Go ahead and embrace your gorgeous-ness and start celebrating…you!

Shall we begin, my friend?

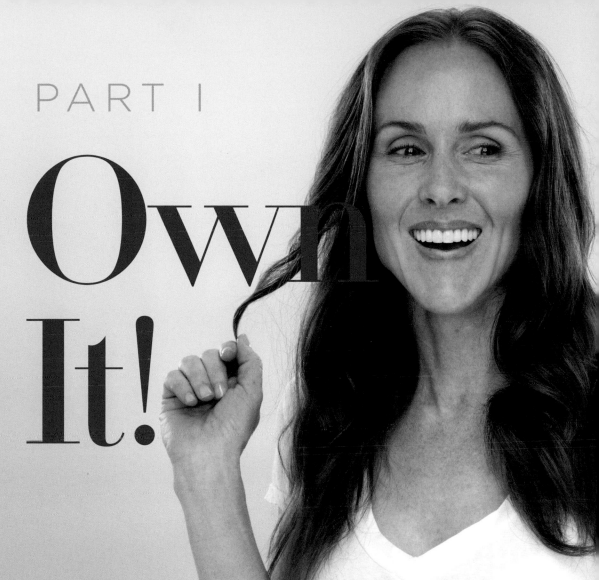

PART I

Own It!

"*What other people think about you*

is none of your business."

— MARILYN MONROE

In this section,
I will help you
discover what a
beautiful woman
you are—
inside and out.

REDEFINING THE
Meaning of True Beauty

This is a book for all the "real women" out there. By real women, I mean women whose career isn't spent in front of the camera and who do not have paparazzi waiting for them when they step out the front door. Women whose busy lives do not include me in their bathroom fixing their hair every morning and whose beauty regimen may not be #1 on their to-do list, because they have so many other responsibilities, but whom I nonetheless consider beautiful. Women just like you. I wrote this book because I want you to embrace just how beautiful you are. I want you to own your beauty and fully accept who you are.

I've waited a long time to share this positive message and take a stand against the current "standard" of beauty that puts incredible pressure on women from all walks of life, from teens and twenty- and thirty-somethings to women in their forties, fifties, sixties, and beyond. That day has come, with this book.

I already share this philosophy with my clients. My goal as a beauty expert is to bring out the best in every woman who sits in my chair—famous or not—by creating a look that not only suits her hair type, lifestyle, and personality but also makes her feel incredibly proud, hold her head up high, and declare her beauty! I always encourage my clients to focus on everything they love about themselves and their looks—not the things they tell me they can't stand. As I once told Nate Berkus on Oprah Radio, it's amazing what happens to a woman when she really takes a moment to look in the mirror and identify with the powerful element of "self" that she already possesses.

The Dangers of "Aspirational" Beauty

I love being a part of the beauty industry and helping women feel great about themselves, but I've also seen its dangerous side and the impossible demands it puts on women to achieve a certain beauty ideal, and the damage that causes.

Many women feel that they've somehow *failed* if they don't fit into the cookie-cutter idea of beauty that the industry has created—if they don't look like the young, airbrushed models and actresses on the covers of magazines and on TV and the silver screen. I think it's a shame that women are criticized in the media if they are not a size 0 with a perfect body, shapely legs that seem to go on forever, a tiny waist, taut, tight abs, chiseled arms, flawless tan skin (sprayed on), and, of course, long perfect hair. I often feel that the beauty industry and the media don't realize the harmful impact this message has on all of us. It may sell magazines and products, but it exacts a terrible price from women when they judge themselves against these standards. Of course they're not fair! Nor are these beauty standards a reality for most women. What about the women out there who have kinky curls or fine, flat hair that won't grow past their shoulders? And what about the average American woman, who is five foot four and a size 14? Or African-American, Latina, Asian, Arab, and Indian women, who are rarely represented in the mainstream beauty industry, if at all?

And let's not forget about the millions of professional women and stay-at-home and working moms out there who simply don't have the time or money to work out with a trainer five days a week and are down on themselves because they've gained a few pounds. It's unrealistic to expect anyone to chase these ridiculous standards. Who has the time? I would rather women be healthy and their best selves, leaving time to enjoy life, and their family and friends.

One of the reasons that women think of themselves as "less than" is because many influential people in the beauty business are sold on the idea of "aspirational beauty," a term I hate. It means that they want you to aspire to be something that you aren't. I ask you, is aspirational beauty better than true beauty? Is a flawless, airbrushed face better than a face with a beautiful smile and well-earned laugh lines? I would love every woman to feel comfortable in her own skin and show the world what a strong, confident, charismatic woman she really is.

The consequences of aspirational beauty are serious. As a result of what the beauty industry and society deem beautiful, women are judged harshly by others and, worst of all, by themselves. Women have told me that they hate the way they look. They tell me they can't even look in the mirror because they are so disgusted with themselves. I, on the other hand, think they look great! Nevertheless, their deep self-loathing carries over to their day-to-day lives, affecting their jobs, relationships, and quality of life.

I was shocked when a twenty-seven-year-old woman told me she thinks she'll never get married because she doesn't look like she just stepped out of the pages of a magazine. What?? That's crazy. But that's how many women think, unfortunately. A thirty-something mother of three told me she refused to go to her class reunion because she didn't look like she did when she was in high school twenty years ago. I thought she looked fantastic.

Comments like these are all too common among women. We live in a society where looks are seemingly everything. As a result, many women equate their self-worth with their looks. That shouldn't be.

My Muse

I am so proud of my mom. I have always thought she looks exotic and different. I remember always wanting darker skin, like she has. (I have been self-tanning since I was in junior high.) My mom's Filipino, Portuguese, and German heritage has blessed her with unique looks. Because of her caramel-colored skin, round face, full nose, and petite frame, she didn't look like any of the other moms when I was going to school in Detroit or, later, in New Baltimore, Michigan. But she was a powerful role model for me because I saw her embrace her looks and love who she is. She still does.

Keep in mind that this wasn't always easy for her. When I was a child, people sometimes questioned or criticized her looks, which I didn't understand. To me, she was the most beautiful woman I had ever seen. I looked at her through the adoring eyes of a child who loves his mother so much. I hated when people made comments about her being too skinny. Then there was the time when someone actually called the house and asked, "Is Tina Turner there? What race is your mother

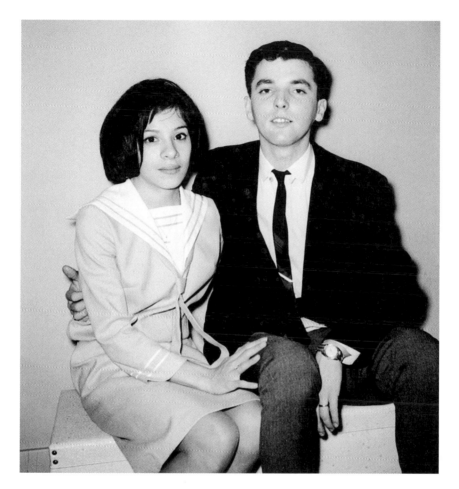

My parents—Helen and Gary, 1960s

exactly?" The tone that the caller used was insulting, but to me the question wasn't insulting in the least. I grew up listening to my mom's idols,
Diana Ross and The Supremes, the Ronettes, and Miss Tina Turner…so
associating the image of these supertalented, beautiful women with my
mother was anything but insulting. It was a compliment. Still, I understood that the caller had a different intention.

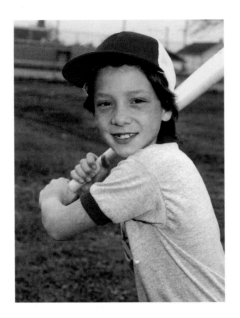

At bat, in 1978

My mom is a superhero to me. She was a selfless wife who, like many women, put her family first, raising three boys. In addition to taking care of my brothers and me, she also worked in factories, at a flower nursery, and even coached my baseball team.

My mom got married when she was very young, so she didn't finish high school until much later, when I was in high school. I admire her for finishing school. She graduated by taking accounting classes. When I opened my salon in Michigan, I made her my manager and accountant. She taught me not to limit myself by what others thought of me.

I remember the magical transformation that took place when my mom would do her hair and makeup for holidays, family functions, or parties she went to with my dad for work. I remember how I would sit outside the door of her half bathroom and watch her get ready. Mom would ask my opinion. (I'd usually tell her to make her hair bigger! Go figure.) I was in awe of those rare moments when it was all about her— even for just a few minutes. I could see how good that made her feel. It literally transformed her. She carried herself differently, standing up tall and confident. People noticed.

What I learned from my mom is that when you accept who you are, ignore other people's opinions, and get rid of that inner voice that reminds you of the flaws you think you have, others will notice, too.

A Worldwide Beauty Epidemic

Clearly, my mom isn't alone. Over the years, many women have told me that they don't feel beautiful because they don't fit into the beauty industry's narrow definition of what they think they "should" look like.

I am so proud of my work on *The Oprah Show* and *The Biggest Loser* and in magazines like *O, The Oprah Magazine* that have allowed me to celebrate real women. Many of the women I had the honor of making over had just given up. They were tired of trying to live up to everyone else's expectations and standards. I began to realize just how much influence the beauty industry has and, therefore, how much responsibility *I* have to help change it.

This was made clear to me again in 2009 while traveling the world with Jessica Simpson to film *The Price of Beauty*, a VH1 docu-series about the lengths to which women go to look beautiful. I was shocked by how much damage this unattainable ideal has actually caused women everywhere. When I came back from the trip, I actually felt embarrassed and ashamed of the industry I've been a part of because its lofty standards have hurt so many women.

It's time to define your own beauty!

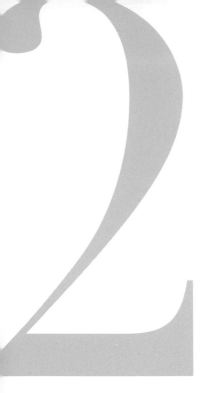

My Story:
FROM THERE
TO HERE
...TO YOU

Although I have been approached to write a book at various times over the last few years, I didn't feel the timing wasn't right. I wasn't ready. I wanted and needed to learn more. Now, at forty-one, after almost twenty years in the industry, I feel I have something substantial to offer.

I've included this chapter for two reasons: First, before I began writing, I reached out to women via social media and asked what you would like to see in this book. Many of you said that you were interested in knowing how I succeeded in my career. The other reason is, in order for me to feel comfortable about giving you my opinions, I need to earn your trust. I want you to know that I did not just arrive at this moment with the wave of a magic wand. The reality is that I've worked really hard to become the best at what I do—and that is to be of service to you.

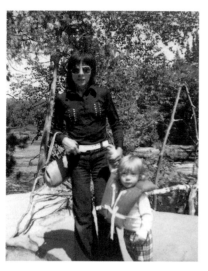

Me and Mom

It All Started With My Mom…

As I've often said, my interest in hairstyling came from an appreciation of my mother and seeing how selflessly she raised my brothers and me. I always wanted to celebrate her and see that she felt as good about herself as she made me feel. In doing so, I realized how interested I was in women's beauty. Soon I was styling hair for my nieces, my sisters-in-law, and my friends. Oh, did I say styling? I should have said "experimenting on!"

A New Path

Originally, I went to college to learn sign language and work with deaf children. During that time, my dad, Gary, retired from his job in the auto industry in Detroit, where he had worked seven days a week, ten to twelve hours a day, often on the night shift, for thirty-two years.

At his retirement party, he said, "Kenney, you are the baby, the last of my three sons, and I want you to be happy. Promise me that thirty-two years from now you will still love whatever career you choose as much as the day you started it."

My dad is a tough man, like Clint Eastwood in *Gran Torino*. He taught us to demand respect and to respect ourselves. He also had me riding a motorcycle at age six…so I didn't

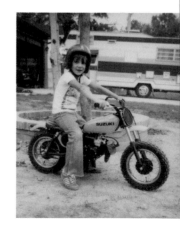

On my motorcycle, age 6

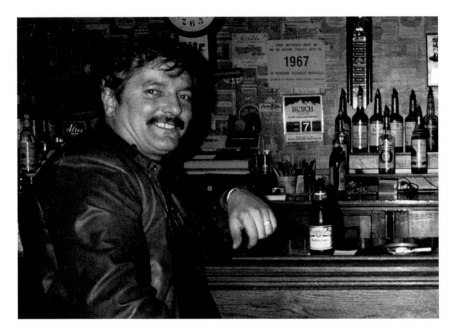

Dad, 1988

know how he'd take it when I told him I wanted to be a hairdresser. His retirement party was at a bar. Everyone had already had a few beers, so I decided there was no better time than the present. I blurted out, "I want to be a hairdresser!"

My dad grabbed me in a headlock, as if he were going to give me a noogie (like guys do when they're goofing around), and said, "Hey, everybody, my kid's gonna be a hairdresser!" Then he bought everyone a round of beer! Like my mom, my dad always taught my brothers and me to believe in ourselves and follow our dreams. He then told me there was no reason to wait for mine. We just needed to find the money for beauty school tuition. My parents were so generous—they cashed in some of their IRAs and my mom took out a loan to cover the costs. I am so grateful for what they did for me. I will never forget it.

I graduated from beauty school in 1994, and it has been a long journey from there to here. It certainly didn't happen overnight.

In the area where I grew up, haircuts with a style cost $8 to $12. (My dad still gets his hair cut near the house where I grew up for $10.) When I finished beauty school, I decided I wanted to go to work on the wealthier side of town in hopes of making more money. I met the owner of a very swanky salon on the west side of town—the more affluent side—through a friend. The owner laughed and said, in a catty tone, that I didn't look like a hairdresser. Maybe she had noticed my tight-rolled jeans, rugged boots, and flan-

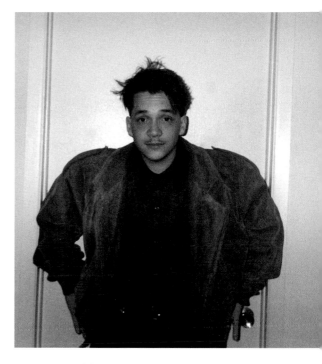

Me, around the same time, in my grunge phase.

nel shirt (grunge was in back then), or maybe it was my nearly jet-black, dyed perm that I'd gel and air-dry until it looked like shellac.

Then I went to another salon where the staff just ignored me and left me standing by myself. I went outside and called my mom, who said, "Are you serious? They're just pretending to be cool—and that's not cool. Go back inside and get that job." After my mom's pep talk, I went back in, asserted myself, and did just that.

The salon was everything I had hoped for, except for the stylist who insisted on calling me "east side rat boy." Oh well, it was a step on the ladder to success. The first step. I was determined to succeed—so determined that I also cleaned the salon at night for extra money.

After a year, I was doing really well. Then I saw a magazine article about an überswanky salon that had just opened in Miami: Oribe, which was, at the time, one of the best (and still is). I felt like I had done everything I could do in Michigan—local fashion shows, photo shoots, and the morning news. Miami was next on my radar. I didn't know anything about Oribe, the owner of the salon, before I read about him, but both he and his career looked glamorous. I had made it this far—what would it hurt to send a résumé?

So I did. No response. I sent another. No response. I sent another and another—maybe ten résumés or more, all with no response. A client of mine then suggested sending a picture of myself in a nice box, since the holidays were approaching. So I sent my résumé again, this time with a picture of me in a beautiful box. I sent it overnight and the next day I received a voicemail and an interview.

So now I had an interview with one of the top salons in the country—and I had nothing to wear. Oh…and I needed a plane ticket, too. My brother Jon was kind enough to put my plane ticket on his credit card for me. Thanks, Jon!

I was still on a very limited budget, but I wanted to look the part (I hoped) of a Miami stylist. I had already made the mistake of not looking the part at the first salon I applied to, so I was not going to do *that* again. I flipped through a men's fashion magazine to see what was in style. I bought some silver satin fabric and had pants made for $7. I bought a Versace winter-thermal shirt that was discounted and on sale. I cut the sleeves off right below the Versace label so that the staff at Oribe would see the name and think I fit in.

But there was one thing I needed that I couldn't fake—Gucci shoes. I had already asked my brother to use his credit card for my plane ticket, so I couldn't ask him for anything more. But I knew whom I could ask. "Mom?" I said. "Come on, mom, I need them. If I don't have them, I won't fit in!" (I know better than that now, which is one of the reasons I'm writing this book.)

My mom and I went to the mall where all the expensive stores were located. You know when you feel uncomfortable but want to act like you know exactly where you're going, so you walk really fast? Well, that's what we did—right up the escalator and past the store (Gucci was on the lower level). I was certain everyone knew we didn't belong there, which of course I later learned probably wasn't true and didn't matter anyway.

When we finally backtracked to the Gucci store, I had an "aha" moment when I saw exactly the same pair of black patent leather loafers I had seen in a magazine—and which I had to wear without socks, of course. I was going by the book this time. I tried not to act too

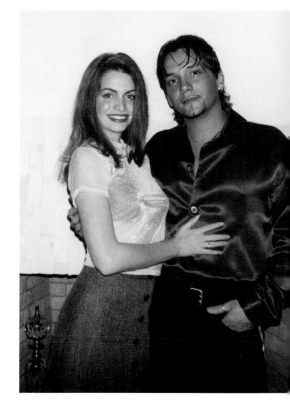

Miami days, 1995

excited, but when I saw those shoes I was convinced the job was mine! (Whatever it takes, right? It's all about thinking positively!)

I flew down to Miami and met with Oribe's manager, a very kind but intimidating man named Omar. We sat on a wooden bench outside the salon, on the porch of a beautiful coral building on Miami's famous Collins Avenue. Within five minutes, Omar offered me the job. I thought, "OK, is this a joke?" remembering the torture I'd endured at the Michigan salons. The difference here was that the people at this salon didn't have to pretend to be cool—they were cool!

Omar invited me in to meet everybody, including Oribe. But when I stood up, my satin pants got snagged on a wood slat in the bench. As I walked away, the snag worsened. I had to tear the thread that was still caught on the bench. One of my pant legs was now shortened to a "Capri pant"—my grand entrance!

I walked inside to an incredibly glamorous and very busy salon. Omar told Oribe I was going to be starting soon. Somehow I felt right at home. We discussed that I would go back to Michigan to gather my things and start working with them in a few months.

I couldn't believe it. Part of the reason I'd come down to Miami was just to challenge and prove to myself that I could do it. And I did! I went back to Michigan, moved in with my parents (at twenty-four), sold my car, and worked as much as possible to save as much money as I could for Miami.

In February 1996, I moved to Florida to start my new job. At the salon, I made very little money as an assistant, but for me it was all about the experience. I quickly ran through my savings. When I got behind on the rent for my apartment, I made extra money cleaning the salon on Sundays, just as I'd done in Michigan, and temping at the front desk. Still, I found it very difficult to make ends meet.

Big, Big Hair…and More Big Hair

Things started to change for me when I met a beautiful young woman at the beach and snuck her into the salon to do her hair on Sundays between cleaning and washing towels. She loved how I did her hair and said she had a "bunch of girlfriends" who would also love what I did. She confided in me that she was, in fact, a stripper and worked at a club just down the street. I soon became the "house mom" at the

Déjà Vu strip club. I did all the girls' hair for free. I worked for tips—and they were great tippers. Most of the girls were students, putting themselves through school, or young women starting their own businesses. They were nothing like you might expect—they were just trying to get by, like I was.

So now I was an assistant at the salon; I worked part-time at the desk and did housekeeping—and I was a "house mom" at a strip club. But now I wanted to do more, so I started to network. I met and began to work with a cool French photographer named Sophie Pangrazzi. Suddenly I found myself doing hair for Sophie's fashion shoots every week. Even so, I was still behind on my rent because I was spending all my money on wigs and hairpieces for Sophie's shoots.

I remember when I got the first copy of a French magazine that showcased our work. Actually, it wasn't exactly a magazine—it was more like a newspaper, similar to the *National Enquirer*, but it had a fashion section and the pictures were gorgeous. It was a start—for both of us, really. Sophie, who was already on her way to success when I met her, went on to become an internationally recognized and awarded photographer. While I wasn't paid to do hair for the shoots, I used the opportunity to collect tear sheets from the magazines where my work was showcased, to build my portfolio.

I started making more contacts—models, photographers, and other people in the business. I still wanted to work more. I knew someone at one of the local high-end hotels, The Astor Place, who agreed to let me start doing fashion shows there on Fridays, during lunch. I begged a local agency to let me work with two of their models for these shows. Since they wouldn't be paid to participate, I promised that I would give them great exposure. So I went and introduced myself to all the local high-end boutiques and got a few to sign on—the Betsy Johnson store was the first to actually lend me clothes. A makeup artist friend agreed to help for free as well. We all needed the exposure! Before the lunch crowd arrived at the hotel, I would close off one of the bathrooms to serve as our hair, makeup, and changing room for the models. It was a single bathroom, but we made it work.

The clothes I was "showing" had already hit the runway six months before, so I would research what the models' hair had looked like on the runway and replicate it. I did this to spread my creative wings and to force myself to learn how to do things I had never done before.

Finally, we were ready. While everyone was eating, we cranked up the music and the two models started strutting through the crowded restaurant. At first, people didn't know what to think. Each girl would come back to our makeshift dressing room and I would change her clothes, just like they do at a real fashion show. Our show lasted all of eighteen to twenty minutes. When we were finished, the crowd applauded. They loved it! We were a hit.

Within a couple of weeks, we were in full swing. Every Friday we put on our Fashion Lunches, and now local fashion television programs and magazines were beginning to cover them. Our shows became quite the scene. For the first time ever, I was recognized for my work, appearing in one of the social pages in *Ocean Drive* magazine. I was so proud. I sent my mom and dad a stack of the magazines, which they still have.

I was now doing a lot of editorial work—hairdressing for models in fashion layouts—in various publications, including *Ocean Drive*, *Fashion Spectrum*, and *Surface Magazine*. I also landed a local agent, Peggy Bremner, who represented hair and makeup artists. She was so good to me. With Peggy's help, I started working more and more.

I got one of my biggest breaks when one of the hairstylists who worked with me at the salon asked me to assist him on a job with model Niki Taylor for CoverGirl. On the morning of the shoot he got sick, so I had to start the hair myself. How nervous was I, prepping the hair of one of the most beautiful women in the world for one of the largest cosmetic companies? I was scared "@!#%-less," but I did my best and everyone was happy.

Niki later called me to style her hair for my first magazine cover ever—for *Ocean Drive*! The national news show, *Fox After Breakfast*, covered the shoot. My mom was a huge fan of the show and always watched. I didn't know they were coming to shoot, so I didn't have time to prep my mom. She nearly fell out of her chair when she saw me on TV, styling Niki Taylor's hair.

Even though I was working nonstop, I was still making "assistant money," doing editorial shoots for magazines and other publications that often paid nothing or very little. I spent more money than I made for each shoot on hairpieces, because I wanted to do the best job I could do.

I was still behind on rent and borrowing my mom's credit card for "it" shoes. My new obsession and must-have shoes were a pair of white patent leather Kenneth Cole loafers. My mom convinced a salesperson at Macy's to take her credit card over the phone for the shoes.

I was now beyond busy doing hair, living near the beach and loving life. One day I was assisting Oribe at work when two of the girls from the strip club came into the salon to visit me. I panicked. Oribe took one look at them and said their hair was "genius." I confessed that I had been doing the girls' hair at night because I was broke. Oribe was intrigued. That night, he took a bunch of the stylists to the club to see what I was up to.

I was creating elaborate hairstyles for the girls, covering them with extensions, and directing them to come onstage with their enormous Brigitte Bardot updos. Then they'd suggestively take out one pin and let their hair fall to their waists. I have to admit, they looked hot doing it. Oribe told me he was impressed and invited me to Paris one week later to assist on couture fashion shows—an amazing learning experience. After the trip, I knew I had to move to New York if I wanted to do real fashion.

New York/L.A.

In New York I focused on doing fashion shoots and editorial. I was still making very little money (in fact, I was nearly stone broke!), but I was getting all the experience I needed.

Along the way, I met Kelli Delaney, a magazine fashion editor at *Allure* and then at *Glamour*. I started off doing hair for small pictures of models in the front of the book. These were not fashion images and were usually only a couple of inches big, but it didn't matter. My name was in the magazine!

I graduated to doing full-page fashion spreads and then magazine covers. At this time models—not celebrities—were photographed for covers. Kelli and I continued to work together for years and she hired me for one of the first celebrity covers I ever did for a major fashion magazine.

Life was good. I really liked working with celebrities. I found them interesting, and I loved living and working in New York.

One day, I received a call at the salon from a hair and makeup agent in Los Angeles, Tnah Louise (now Di Donato, my godson Nicolai's mother). She had attended a recent fashion show in Los Angeles and saw a model on the runway whose hair I had cut in New York City. She loved the cut and tracked me down. She offered to represent me in Los Angeles and asked if I was interested. I said no...I had no interest whatsoever in leaving New York, but I really liked her. We spoke three more times before I agreed to take a trip to L.A. to meet her.

I had the opportunity to do an advertising shoot with Kathy Ireland in Los Angeles around the same time that Tnah called me again to see if I wanted to stay with her in L.A. and "see what she could do for me." It was now brutally cold in New York. Did I mention that she had a pool?

I went to L.A., booked as a "local hairstylist," for the Kathy Ireland job. Tnah picked me up from the airport and took me to her house, where I met her two-year-old son, Romeo, and roommate, Tip (whom you'll meet later in this book). They kindly gave me a futon to sleep on in the living room. I was so grateful.

Whenever I had to go to Santa Barbara to work with Kathy, Tnah let me take her car. Later, Tnah would rent a (not so cool) seafoam green Ford Aspire for me. At the time, Tip was a model agent in the same office where Tnah worked. I ended up staying in Los Angeles for two months during my first visit. I was hooked. They lived in the Hollywood Hills, had magical views, and the weather was warm! Tnah sent me to meet a lot of people in those two months, but really I didn't do much hairstyling (except for Tnah and Tip whenever they needed it). I stayed busy cleaning the house, shopping for groceries, cleaning the pool, and doing laundry. One day, I painted Tip's bathroom a whimsical, washed blue and glued stars on the ceiling to remind her of where she grew up in Hawaii.

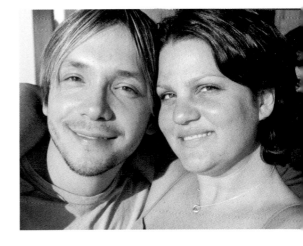

With Tip

I went back to work in New York for just a month before returning to L.A. The meet-and-greets Tnah had sent me on paid off. Not only was I working every couple of months doing advertising with Kathy Ireland (which I would go on to do for years), but Tnah told me she had booked me to work in L.A. with several new celebrity clients.

Jessica

Between celebrity magazine covers and fashion spreads in New York, and the work Tnah was sending me in L.A., I was getting around.

On a trip back to New York in 1999, Charlie Walk, one of my clients (an executive at Sony's Columbia Records, who went on to become the president of Sony's Epic record label, and now heads Charlie Walk Entertainment), asked me to go to Los Angeles to do a shoot with one of his brand-new artists. I had to decline his offer because of other work commitments. A little while later, Tnah called from Los Angeles and asked if I could come back to work with a new Columbia recording artist. I told her I wasn't able to, but wondered if she was talking about the same artist Charlie had mentioned.

Soon after, Charlie called me again about his new artist, Jessica Simpson. Her first album cover shoot was coming up and she needed to be photographed with long hair. The problem was that the hairstylist who had previously done Jessica's hair bleached it and cut it short. I was working with some other Columbia recording artists, so Charlie was aware of my work with extensions and asked me if I could help. On a flight from New York to L.A., I sewed Jessica's hair extensions (freshly colored by master colorist Rita Hazan). When I ran out of thread, I got a fresh supply from one of the flight attendants. However, the thread was from a hotel sewing kit and was all different colors, from blue, green, and yellow to red, white, black, and brown. (I pointed this out to Jessica when I met her the next day.) I got some strange looks while I sewed Jessica's extensions that night on the plane, since my own hair at the time was exactly the same shade of blonde. I'm certain some of the other passengers thought the hair was for me and that I might walk off the plane as a woman . . . with facial hair!

The next day, when I met Jessica, she showed me a picture of what her hair looked like "before." She asked if I could make it look like that again. When I was finished, I remember her looking into the mirror and telling me her hair looked exactly like it did "before"!

Our fate was sealed. By this time, I had worked with several other recording artists. *But* the moment I lay on the floor, blowing Jessica's newly lengthened golden locks with two hair dryers—as the camera started clicking and her single "I Wanna Love You Forever" was cued up—I was smitten. I was blown away by the voice that came out of this petite, soft-spoken young Texan, wearing a pink leather jacket styled by renowned fashion stylist Rachel Zoe (whom I'd first met and worked with back in my Miami days) and holding a vintage microphone. She could really belt it out! Jessica is sweet, funny, beautiful, and the girl can sing, I mean *sing*! It was a great day, the pictures turned out amazing, I had made a new friend, and I knew we would be seeing a lot more of each other.

Home Sweet Hollywood

I began to work more and more in Los Angeles but kept going back and forth between coasts. My good friend from New York, Cheri Oteri, now had a place in Los Angeles too. We used to drive around Los Angeles in Cheri's Toyota Paseo, and I would scream out of the car at people, "Simmer down now!" Cheri later incorporated this phrase in one of her most famous skits on *Saturday Night Live*, when she played Nadine, the counter girl at Burger Castle who would hilariously order customers to "simmer down now!"

I was still staying with Tnah and Tip, but thought it was time to get an apartment of my own. Cheri and I found one a block away from her place. I loved L.A., but remained bicoastal. I continued to work with new celebrities as I built my résumé. I knew that a permanent move to Los Angeles was inevitable, though, and I finally made that move in 2000. I would go on to work with Christina Applegate, Milla Jovovich, Lucy Liu, Alyssa Milano, Lindsay Lohan, Minnie Driver, Jennifer Lopez, Anne Hathaway, Brittany Murphy, Hilary Swank, Renee Zellweger, Anne Heche, Cameron Diaz, Nicole Richie, Amanda Peete, Pamela Anderson, Carmen Electra, Holly Hunter, Camryn Manheim, Kate Beckinsale, Felicity Huffman, Marcia Cross, Michelle Williams, Megan Fox, Kirsten Dunst, Debra Messing, Heather Locklear, Denise Richards, Calista Flockhart and many more.

Then things got really busy. Once, while living in L.A., I did six actresses' hair for one award show—Kristen Davis, Michael Michelle, Portia de Rossi, Lara Flynn Boyle, Sela Ward, and Kim Cattrall. I was crazy in those days. I never said no!

My First Salon

In 2002, I opened my first salon outside of my hometown in Michigan and asked my parents to run it. My mom and dad manage the salon better than I could have ever imagined. They run it like I would, only more organized! The salon is just like me: it's small, not necessarily from the cool side of town, but has a heart of gold and is capable of great things. The stylists at the Ken Paves Salon in Michigan have traveled the world with me, worked with my biggest clients, and assisted me with many of the makeover shows I have done. I am very proud of where I came from, and the Ken Paves Salon in Michigan reflects that pride.

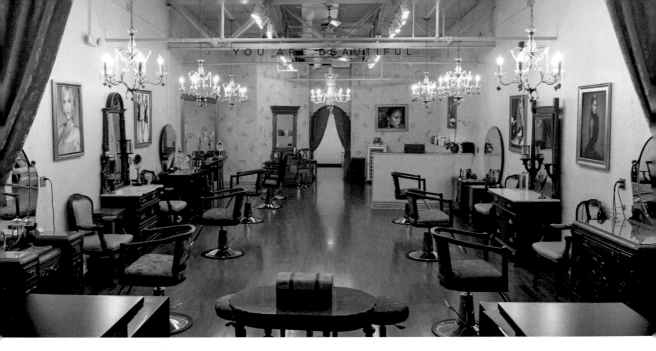

The Ken Paves Salon in Michigan.

Enter Oprah

2003 was a big year for me. I appeared on *The Oprah Winfrey Show* for the first time in May. I have to say, there's nothing like hearing one of your greatest idols say your name. That would be *big* for anyone, but for me it was epic and beyond imaginable. Having my work validated by Oprah Winfrey made me believe in myself as a stylist and, more importantly, that I had value as a person—and that I had something to share with the world. You have to understand that my mom and I were diehard fans from the moment *The Oprah Winfrey Show* went national in 1986. You've gotten to know us in the previous pages, so you can imagine how well we related to everyone and every story on *The Oprah Winfrey Show*. Oprah campaigned for the underdog, and made me feel like it was OK to be me, long before I met her. She made me feel like I could do anything if I believed in myself. She put herself out there as living proof. I never thought in a million years Oprah would tell me that I help other people realize they are worth being their best. After all, that is what she did for me. Not to mention that she called me the big kahuna of Hollywood hair! I worked with Oprah and *The Oprah Winfrey Show* from 2003 until it ended in 2011, loving every second of it. I still work for the magazine and have appeared on OWN, her Oprah Winfrey Network.

To Extend or Not To Extend? Extend!

At this point in my career, extensions and attention-grabbing hair transformations are my forte, but then, they had always gone under the radar, leaving everyone wondering, "Did she cut her hair? Did she color her hair? Is her hair longer than it was?"

By now I had been working with Jessica Simpson for a few years, and her hair was the topic of much conversation among the executives at her record label. They insisted that I keep her hair long and straight because that was what all the other blonde pop stars were doing at the time. For Jessica's first music video, Rachel Zoe and I had another idea—to make her hair wavy, a look that has now become her signature style. We filmed Jessica, with her new waves, for an entire day, a departure that got me into a lot of trouble with the executives in New York when an assistant on the set sent them an image of Jessica's new look. We had to reshoot. This time Jessica's hair was perfectly straight.

When it was time for MTV's Video Music Awards in August 2003, Jess and I had enough. She was now ready to experiment with her hair, just as so many of my other clients were doing. For the VMAs, Jessica's mom, Tina, dressed her in a gorgeous, white, low-cut Armani suit. I did not see this look with long straight hair. I custom made a Marilyn Monroe (above the shoulder) half-wig for Jess to wear with the suit. It looked amazing. She said she felt like a different woman. When reporters on the red carpet asked if she had cut her hair, Jess did what Jess does best—she said exactly what was on her mind, blurting out, "I didn't cut my hair. I'm wearing a wig!" Only Jess!

Some clients' publicists made me swear that I would never mention that *their* clients wore extensions or hairpieces. It was still taboo at the time. But Jessica and I would change all that with the VMAs that year. Jess loved the freedom that wigs, extensions, and hairpieces gave her, and we started to transform her look from moment to moment. A hair icon was born!

Celine

More good things were to come in 2003, when a friend of mine, Sammy Mourabit, with whom I had worked in Miami around the time I met Rachel Zoe, and who traveled with Celine Dion as her makeup artist, called to tell me that he had given my name to the designers of Cirque du Soleil and its creator Franco Dragone, to consider me for the job of head hair designer for a new show they were doing with Celine Dion in Las Vegas. I met with the design team in Los Angeles and discussed what they were looking for. They wanted someone who had experience working with wigs and extensions. I got the job and was the hair designer for Celine Dion's "A New Day," her long-running Las Vegas show. I moved to Las Vegas for six months to work with Celine and the show's dancers for the beginning of the show, and I continued to go back, occasionally, throughout its run.

Celine is amazing. Such a professional. I learned so much from her. I styled her hair for the show, for appearances, several music videos, magazine shoots, and even for the book she did with Anne Geddes, *Miracle: A Celebration of New Life*. I will always adore Celine, whom I met when her hair was long, right before she had it cut very short and dyed it blonde. Although I did not cut her hair short or color it, I supported Celine for doing what made her feel good. However, I remember all the nasty blogs and comments from some of her fans, who thought I had cut her long hair short. There was even a website with a doctored picture of me wearing a pair of devil horns, presumably for cutting Celine's hair too short! I continued to work with Celine as she transitioned back to her long brown hair.

The show was going well and I started to do a lot more with Celine. I traveled with her to New York for the daytime talk shows and was even with her when she received her star on the Hollywood Walk of Fame. I would fly back and forth on Southwest Airlines from Vegas to L.A., sometimes every other day, to take care of my other clients.

Branching Out

In 2004, I launched my first line of hair-care products. Previously, I had been a spokesperson for Pantene and Johnson & Johnson. Scented with 100 percent essential oils, Paves Professional was a sulfate-free line before sulfate-free products became popular. I won many awards that year in the cosmetic industry for this revolutionary new line, including Breakthrough Product of the Year at the Cosmetic Executive Women (CEW) Beauty Insider's Choice Awards. Later, I became Chrysler's convertible season spokesperson with my "Convertible Proof" hairspray. Yes, I said Chrysler.

All About… Eva

That same year—in 2004—the television show *Desperate Housewives* premiered. I was an instant fan. I especially loved the character of Gabrielle Solis, played by Eva Longoria (the only person I've ever asked to work with). After the show had aired, I saw Eva in an interview, and she seemed like a kind and compassionate person, someone I would like to work with. Plus I wanted to get my hands on her hair!

Shortly after seeing Eva's interview, I received a phone call about styling her hair for a magazine cover. I was over the moon! I couldn't wait.

Well, as it turned out, I would have to wait. Apparently Eva's publicist already had another hairdresser in mind, and the magazine would use that person. I understood that, of course: I appreciate loyalty. Then I received another request, this time from a photographer friend, to work with Eva. Same story: I would have to wait. Eva's publicist said they already had a hairdresser. By the time this happened to me for a third time, everyone around me knew how badly I wanted to work with Eva.

Not long afterward, I was booked to do makeovers for *The Oprah Winfrey Show*. A very good friend of mine, Ellen Rakieten, who was the executive producer of the show, asked if I wanted to enlist any of my "celeb" clients to help me with the makeover. Funny she should ask, because I knew that Oprah had just interviewed the cast of *Desperate Housewives*. This was my in! I replied that I would be happy to ask Jessica Simpson and Lara Flynn Boyle to be on Oprah's show. Then I explained the whole Eva story and asked Ellen if she would mind asking Eva to do a makeover with me. (Seriously, if that's not pulling out the big guns, I don't know what is.) I thought for sure this was it…me and Eva, finally. But Ellen explained that because *Desperate Housewives* was filming in Los Angeles, Eva could not travel to Chicago for the makeover show. Jessica and Lara, however, appeared on *Oprah* with me.

Fast forward to July 28, 2005: My best bud, Jessica Simpson, was premiering her huge movie, *The Dukes of Hazzard*, and I was going to style her hair and attend the premiere. Jessica looked amazing that night and she was great in the movie. Also, I heard that Eva Longoria was in the building! When I bumped into Eva Mendes, who knew, like Jess, how badly I wanted to meet Eva Longoria, she said she would introduce me to her.

(One thing you may not know about me is that I am very shy, believe it or not. Now, Eva Longoria's nickname for me is "shivering Chihuahua," which describes me perfectly whenever I go somewhere and don't know a lot of people. I guess I sit in the corner alone and shiver, while she's always like, "Kenney, get over here!")

Back to the story: So as Eva Mendes and I were walking over to meet Eva Longoria, who was standing with another mutual friend, Wilmer Valderrama, Eva walked up to me and said, "Hi, I'm Eva, and I'm a big fan of your work. I'd love to work with you one day." I was in shock!

Now this part, unfortunately, is not made up: I literally turned around and walked away—without saying a word. I have no idea to this day what I was thinking. I actually walked over to the bar with Wilmer, got a drink, and ran to find Jessica for backup. I told her, "OK. I totally just messed up, but at the after party you have to help me talk to Eva." Jess just laughed because she knows how shy I can be, but Eva never showed up at the after party.

My luck changed a month later. In August, the MTV Video Music Awards were held in Miami Beach, and I was there working with Jessica. Later that night, when I was hanging out at an after party with Jess, Paulina Rubio, Ashlee Simpson, and some other friends, I looked up and saw Eva walk into the room. This is where I sound crazy: I jumped over a couch that was in front of me, ran up to Eva, sat her down, and said, "Oh my God, I am so sorry and so embarrassed I didn't say anything to you when we met. I'm really shy, and I think you are so great—and I would love to do your hair!" I'm sure I said way more. I had verbal diarrhea.

Eva, in true form, said, "God, honey, I would love that. You can do my hair for the Emmy Awards next month." Eva is a woman of her word. I did in fact do her hair for the Emmys the following month. I arrived at her house an hour early to set up all my equipment. Anyone who knows me knows I am always late. This was a first for me. I brought lights, a mirrored vanity, and every hair tool, hairpiece, product, comb, and brush I owned. I took over Eva's dining room while she made huevos rancheros for breakfast.

One last thing: After Eva left for the Emmys and I was packing up all my equipment, I noticed I had burned a big hole in her wooden dining room table. I saw her later that night at an Emmy after party and confessed that I'd burned her table. Eva said, "Oh, honey, that's fine, I love my hair." We've worked together steadily ever since.

Getting Wiggy

In 2005 I also patented the design of the hairpieces I had created and was using on all my clients, including the short, Marilyn Monroe bob-style wig Jessica wore to the MTV Video Music Awards in 2003. Later, in 2006, Jessica and I launched my line of HairDo extensions.

At the same time, I continued to work with all my clients, styling them for television, magazines, and the red carpet, while designing looks for plays and movies. I even made a screen debut in *The Wedding Planner*, with Jennifer Lopez (I did her hair for the movie). She and director Adam Shankman gave me a scene in the movie where I deliver pizza. I also appeared in Jessica's movie *Blonde Ambition*, where I designed her look and played myself.

Because of the exposure I was getting on *The Oprah Winfrey Show*, I started to do even more on-camera work for *Extreme Makeover*, *America's Next Top Model*, *E!*, Style Network, and many others. I won a slew of awards for my work—and the media were giving me titles like "Hottest Hairdresser in Hollywood." How cool is that? Not bad for a kid from Detroit (the Motor City)!

New Beginnings

2005 was a big year for me in other ways, too. I was taping a TV hair segment in Los Angeles and had rented a second-story salon to do the filming, since I didn't own a salon in L.A. My then assistant, Tip, ran downstairs to pluck a rose from the garden of a beautiful, quaint cottage next door. After the shoot was over, she came back with a glorious rose in her hair. She told me that the cottage was actually a salon and that I had to go take a look and meet the owner.

From the moment I saw it, the cottage reminded me of my salon in Michigan. It was unassuming but filled with charm. By now, everyone who worked at the cottage salon had left for the day—except for the owner, Jordan Schwartz. He greeted me with the kindest eyes and smile. Jordan was eccentric—and fabulous! He looked like the coolest cat that had just arrived from London in the Swinging Sixties! We sat and talked for hours in the beautiful garden outside the salon.

Near the end of our conversation Jordan told me that he had been asking for an angel to come and take over his salon in the way he had dreamed. He said he thought that angel was me. Jordan told me he was sick—he had cancer—and had yet to tell his staff that he was looking to sell, because he was unsure of his health. At the time, I really was not looking for a salon in Los Angeles, but for some reason I said

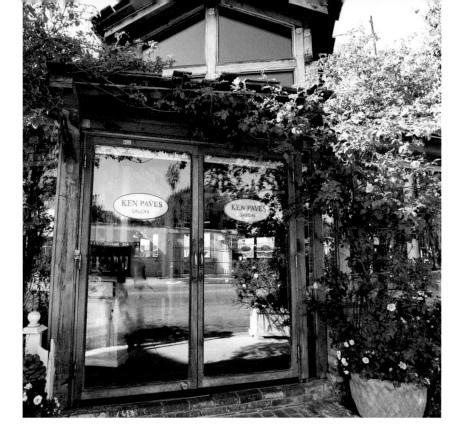

The salon in L.A.

to Jordan, "I think it is me—I'll take over the salon under one condition: You stay!"

Jordan said this was his condition, too. We almost had a deal. As it turned out, my mom just happened to be in town and we agreed that if she liked it, Jordan and I would have a deal! The next day I went to the salon with my mom and my friends Ellen Rakieten and Nate Berkus.

My mom had the final say, and I brought Nate along because I wanted to pick his brain for decorating ideas. When we walked in, the salon was busy, unlike the day before. A woman there said, "Those two guys are on Oprah." Jordan turned to me and asked, "Should I know you? Are you somebody?" I said, "No. Sometimes I do makeovers on Oprah."

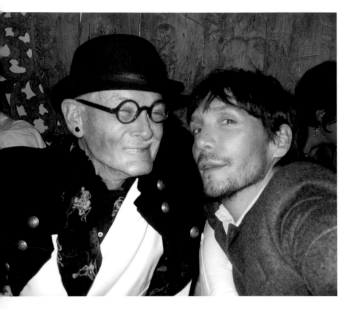

Jordan and me

I knew then for sure that this was meant to be. When Jordan had asked me to take over his salon the previous day, he didn't know anything about me or my career—he had chosen me just for who I am. My mom said she loved the cottage, and Nate said I needed to make it look like something out of *Town and Country* magazine, with a little Chanel and some Tiffany blue thrown in. That is exactly what I did and how the Ken Paves Salon West Hollywood came to be.

Jordan continued to work with and inspire us until his passing in March 2010. My favorite story about Jordan goes back to when I was doing makeovers for *America's Next Top Model*. The producers chose a specific photo of the 1960s supermodel Jean Shrimpton for one of the makeovers. I knew it was the perfect cut for Jordan to do, and I asked him if he would do it. The producers then asked me if I was sure Jordan could do the cut, because by this time his hands were shaking quite a bit. I said yes, and when they asked Jordan himself, he hesitantly answered that he was sure he could do it, because he had actually cut Jean Shrimpton's hair for the same photo the producers were using as a reference—a very cool moment.

I went on to sell my products on HSN in 2006 and moved to QVC in 2009. I am grateful that I have had success with my products on QVC around the world ever since. My lovely mother has traveled the world with me and appeared with me on QVC. People love her—which makes me very happy.

Victoria

In November 2006, I was at the Hassler Hotel in Rome, styling Jennifer Lopez's hair for the wedding of Tom Cruise and Katie Holmes, when there was a delicate knock on the door. A petite, beautiful, fresh-faced woman entered the room. It was Victoria Beckham. The first thing she said was "Wow. That is a lot of hair." I had filled the room with hair extensions to create any of the looks Jennifer could possibly want. I remember Victoria as very soft-spoken and polite, with a great smile—and incredibly poised and chic!

A year later, in 2007, after David and Victoria Beckham had moved to Los Angeles, Victoria told her management, "I want the hair-dresser I met in Rome who had all that hair." It would take some time for Victoria and me to coordinate our schedules, but in the meantime she worked with someone else whom I'd recommended.

I was thrilled at the prospect of working with Victoria. Eva Longoria and I were both Spice Girl fans. Well, I was actually more of a Victoria fan because of her fashion, style, and hair! The next time I actually saw Victoria was in 2008, when Eva and I were together in London and flew to Manchester for a Spice Girl concert. I had provided Victoria and some of the other girls in the group with some of my products and had arranged to have one of my hairdress-ers style their hair for the tour. Eva and I were escorted backstage to Victoria's dressing room to say hi before the show started—and we instantly hit it off. Not only does Victoria have a wicked fashion sense, she also has a wicked sense of humor. Victoria has become one of my dearest friends. She has inspired me in many ways, most obviously as a fashion icon but also as an amazing mother, wife, and kind spirit. Victoria has always encouraged me not to limit myself by what anyone else expects of me, but to design my own destiny.

A Journey I Could Never Have Imagined

Also in 2008, my peers from across the nation elected me for a Hairdressers Unlocking Hope Award, a philanthropic award that means a great deal to me.

In 2009, I went on an incredible journey around the world with Jessica Simpson and Cacee Cobb for the VH1 documentary series *The Price of Beauty* to discover how the rest of the world defines beauty. The trip was eye-opening for all of us. Even though other countries have different ideas of beauty than America does, the pressure to conform to those beauty standards is still all too present. The series ended with a fashion show that represented the beauty of women from all around the globe. It was magnificent.

In 2010 I started doing makeovers for NBC's hit, *The Biggest Loser*—and have just finished filming my fifth season with the show. I am so proud of the work I have done with this extraordinary show. We need more positive television programs like it that inspire and give us hope that it is never too late to become our best self.

Disney Magic

In 2009 I also received a phone call that I would never have imagined—from Disney! Peggy Holmes, the director of a new animated Disney Fairies film, *Secret of the Wings*, explained that Disney was introducing a new Fairy character and she wanted me to design her hair.

Disney! I believe in Disney magic. I tried to act as cool as I could be on the phone and hoped Peggy Holmes wouldn't hear my voice trembling with excitement. As happy as I was to talk to her, all I could think about was hanging up and three-way calling my parents and my niece Chloe to let them know. I am beyond honored and humbled to be a part of the Disney family. When I was a child, my father worked seven days a week to provide for his family. One year, he saved up all his vacation

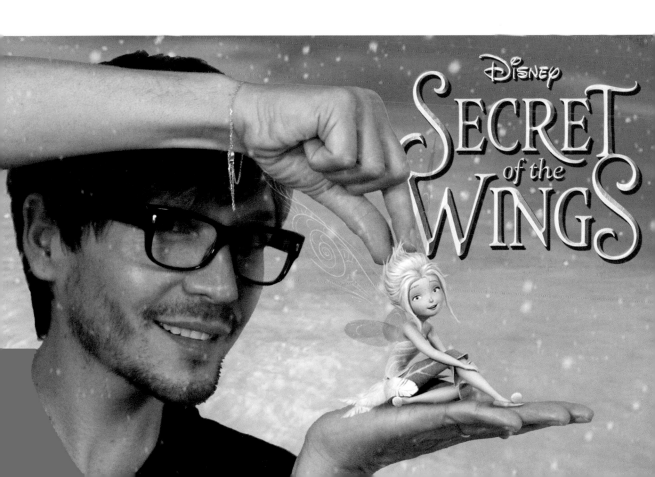

days and drove our motor home down to Florida so that we could visit Walt Disney World Resort. There is nothing like Disney magic, and to this day, I remember that trip.

The thing I loved the most about the phone conversation with Peggy was her honesty. She let me know that I was not the only person Disney was considering for the job, but she was intrigued by my philanthropic work with children. She wanted to work with a hairstylist who shared Disney's passion and imagination. We hit it off and I was hired to design the hair for Periwinkle, a brand-new Fairy.

Shortly after my conversation with Peggy, I was invited to Walt Disney Studios to meet with the director, producers, and animators who magically bring these characters to life. Of course, I brought Tip, who was equally excited about the project. I felt like a child again—I was in awe of the artistry of the animation stills we were shown. I felt humbled by the beauty of the work and hoped that mine would be good enough.

The day I created Periwinkle's hair was true magic. I worked with a live model who resembled the character in a room that had "winter woods" as the backdrop. Every move I made was photographed and videoed. I was nervous but also excited. When I was finished, Periwinkle was born. She had a cool, short, cropped pixie hairstyle. I looked outside the wall of glass where I had been working at all the people whose imagination had created Periwinkle, and I could see in their eyes that she was alive!

My partnership with Disney took another turn in 2010 when, without any explanation, I was asked to come back to the Disney offices in Burbank. I imagined it was to touch up Periwinkle's wig, so I asked Tip to meet me there with my styling kit.

When we arrived at a boardroom for our meeting, I found out that the Disney team wanted to discuss the opportunity of creating a Disney Fairy personal care product line in my name. I was speechless.

I immediately said yes. After all, I had grown up enthralled by Disney productions and found magic and hope in all of their programming. In researching the fairies to create Periwinkle's look, I had come to learn even more about how relevant and important the Disney Fairy message is to our young girls, especially with all the negative influences they face today. The Disney Fairies are all about individuality, talent, and kindness. This is what is considered beautiful in the Fairy world, just as it is in mine. I was so proud to develop Ken Paves for Disney, inspired by Tinker Bell and her fairy friends, because this line represents the exact message I am trying to communicate to the world, which is that we are all unique and beautiful in our own ways and that true beauty is a measure of the value we place on ourselves and others as human beings.

Self Help

Recently I launched a new product line, called Self Help Care of Ken Paves, based on the needs I have seen in women—from my mom and other family members to my friends and even my celebrity clients. I got the idea for Self Help Hair Care when I was doing makeovers for women on *The Oprah Winfrey Show* and noticed how extremely damaged their hair was. I always start working with a woman by addressing the condition of her hair—so this is important to me. I wanted to create Self Help so that women can makeover their own hair at home, without me or an expensive salon. As with my Disney line, the philosophy behind Self Help Care is that women are already beautiful—all on their own—and it's time to celebrate that.

The X Factor

In 2011, my good friend Charlene (who is pictured in this book) called me and said she had mentioned me to her friend Jeff Burroughs, the head of commercial development for Syco Television (Simon Cowell's company) and also brand manager for *The X Factor*. Syco was bringing *The X Factor* to the United States and looking for top beauty experts to bring the contestants on the show to the next level.

Jeff and I met to discuss the show and hit it off instantly. He said Simon Cowell's idea was to also focus on the hair and makeup artists who help to turn the contestants into superstars. That was exactly the kind of project I wanted to be part of. I had spent 18 years doing this already. Everyone seems to forget the transformation that so many artists undergo on the way up, believing instead that they were born as full-blown, superstylized stars. *The X Factor* would allow people to meet the contestants, most of whom look just like the viewers themselves and then watch everything that goes into creating brandable megastars—stars in the making who compete for $5 million on *The X Factor* stage! What interested me is that Jeff said they wanted to find atists who represented everyone watching at home. That was exactly what I wanted to do.

However, my superbusy schedule and other contractual obligations

> I LOVE INSPIRING AND MAKING people feel good about themselves, and I continue to appear on more and more television shows as a beauty expert. I have also started producing beauty-related television shows, which brings me back to the purpose of this book: to give women a positive message about defining their own beauty.

made it impossible for me to do *The X Factor*. We went round and round, talking with studio heads, lawyers, and others, and still couldn't find a way to make it work. Simon Cowell, however, wanted to meet with me. He and I hit it off automatically. I do think he is a genius with a wicked sense of humor, and my dad –yes, my dad—is his biggest fan. He loves that "cocky" and wears a T-shirt every day, just like he does. (Thanks a lot, Simon. Mom and I cannot get my dad into anything but a T-shirt. His excuse is, "Hey, come on. My boy Simon does it!")

Simon asked why I was so open to do this. I said, "Honestly, Simon, no one else could do it like I can." I went on to explain that I had worked with some great popular music stars and acts, including Jennifer Lopez, Eve, the Dixie Chicks, Taylor Swift, Lady Gaga, Britney Spears, Avril Lavigne, Paulina Rubio, Jessica and Ashlee Simpson, LeAnn Rimes, Mindy McCready, Marc Anthony, Anastasia, Christina Milian, Mandy Moore, Fergie, Alejandro Sanz, Renée Fleming, and many more. But I also told him that I had the one thing most other stylists don't have: a knack for making "real" people into their own stars. My work with *The Oprah Winfrey Show* helped me to perfect my skill at turning people who feel their looks are ordinary at best into megawatt versions of themselves. One of Simon's executives said she had seen every *Oprah* show I had done and was a huge fan of my work.

There was a lot more back and forth between lawyers, managers, and others. . . with no resolution. But I wanted to do the show, so I did it on blind faith, without a contract. I knew I had to be there. I'm glad I did.

3

SOME OF THE
Real Women
in My Life

Before we go any further, I would like to introduce you to thirteen real women in my life—good friends and family members—whom I've invited to come along on this journey. These are women whose lives are perhaps more similar to yours than the women shown in ads and commercials, on magazine covers, and on the red carpet, but who nonetheless represent true beauty to me, just as you do.

I wanted to begin with photographs of each of these fabulous women looking natural—sans makeup, with their hair down and wearing white T-shirts—to show how beautiful they are *by just being*. This book is all about accepting and enhancing your natural beauty, and I want everyone to look at each of the women in this book and say, "Hey! She's wearing a white T-shirt. She isn't done up. But she looks beautiful! So I must look beautiful, too."

My mom, Helen,

inspired me to write this book. At four foot eleven and three-quarters, she is petite but powerful. Growing up, we had a measuring wall in the basement because my older brothers, Chris and Jon, and I (three crazy, wisecracking boys) always wanted to know how tall we were. We also measured mom, who was a good sport about all this. She would say she was five feet tall and we'd always shout, "No, you're four eleven!"

I want to be sure to get her height right in this book, because she wasn't too happy when I accidentally told Nate Berkus on Oprah's radio show that she's four foot one—a comment that also made it onto Oprah.com (Sorry, mom!) I really didn't realize I said she was four foot one until she showed me the interview online. Well, after all these years, I have to say, Chris and Jon, listen up: I recently went with mom to a doctor's appointment, where she was measured, and yes, she is five feet tall! Does she always have to be right?

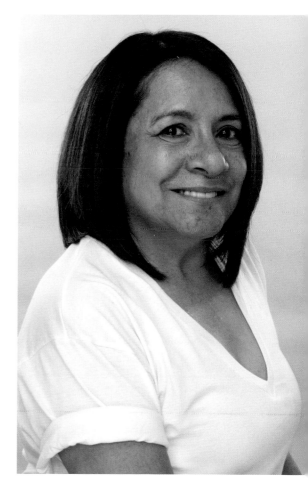

Helen was the kind of mom who was always there for us. She took time to make my favorite dinner—lasagna—and drove me wherever I needed to go—the movies, the mall, or bowling with my friends. She also coached my baseball team. "Heck, yeah," says my mom. "They needed a coach. I was there. I was a tomboy when I was growing up. When I was in high school, I played on the varsity baseball and basketball teams. People always asked me how I could possibly be a forward on my basketball team, and a good one at that. I might not have been tall, but I was quick. I would simply run around much taller opponents—and I could hit a baseball as far as any boy could. So it was a pleasure to coach Ken's team."

My mom even helped me rebuild my first car. When I was fourteen, my brother Jon brought home a '68 Mustang. Mom and I instantly became mechanics. I would save money from collecting returnable cans and mom would help out with extra money from her part-time job to buy parts for the car. So there we were, the two of us, in our garage, covered in grease, taking the car apart. Believe it or not, we replaced the carburetor, the brakes, and the entire interior. We even put new fenders on the car. If we didn't know what we were doing, we figured it out together.

Helen and I drove around all the time. Once I got my permit, there was no stopping us. Some of the best times we had were when we drove to a junkyard for old Mustang parts, about 40 miles from home. Mom and I would jump in the car, singing everything from Diana Ross to Air Supply—all the way there and back.

My mom has always been so encouraging and supportive, telling me that I can do anything I set my mind on. Some of her friends would ask why she let me drive her around all the time. She just shrugged and said, "I trust him. This is the way he is going to learn." Her words and positive attitude are what helped me develop the self-assurance and strength to become successful later in life.

In fact, my mom and my dad would always tell me and my brothers that we could do whatever we wanted to, as long as we worked hard for it. I never forgot that. When I was a teenager and a budding hairstylist, my mom always encouraged me to follow my dreams, despite all the lopsided haircuts I gave her—and the many perms I forgave her for giving me! My mom was definitely a kitchen hairstylist.

"I would tell Ken and my other sons, 'Whatever you want to do, just go for it,'" says Helen. "I also told them, 'Don't let anybody tell you that you can't do something, because you can do anything you want to do.'"

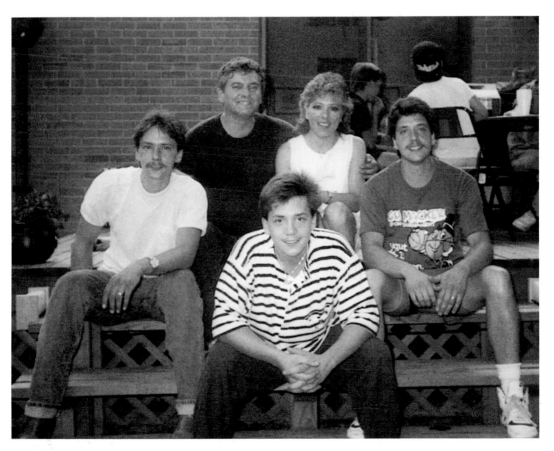

My family in the 1980s

If you ever meet my longtime friend, **Tip,** you will pass out from the positive energy she exudes and the way she carries herself. Tip radiates and captivates…she is truly beautiful. I call her "Flippa" because she is always fluttering and buzzing about, sharing love and light with everyone around her. She shares the same love with herself and it shows.

I met Tip when I first came to L.A., and she has worked with me ever since. Tip now works with me in my Los Angeles salon and has met everyone, in our travels, from Lady Gaga and Jennifer Lopez to Oprah. Some people might feel intimidated, meeting superstars like this. Not Tip. She walks into the room and says, almost singing, "Hi, ladies! You look lovely." When they ask, "What's going on?" she says, "Everything!" Anyone who meets Tip instantly feels comfortable because she's so comfortable in her own skin. Tip's positive vibe is contagious. She's always happy. Tip finds the best part of any situation and the good in everyone. She has the confidence to go anywhere she wants to go by herself—the beach, dinner, a movie. She recently traveled to Honduras on a ten-day trip all by herself.

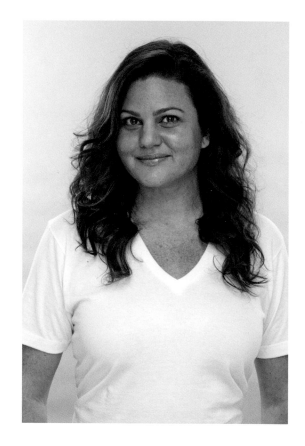

Tip has lots of friends, but she also has a passion for life. She doesn't depend on anyone else. I envy that about her. Are you kidding me? I'm one of those people who can't walk to the bathroom alone in a crowded room. Tip has walked to the bathroom with me a million times. She has also been there for me in my most difficult and my greatest moments. Thanks, Tip.

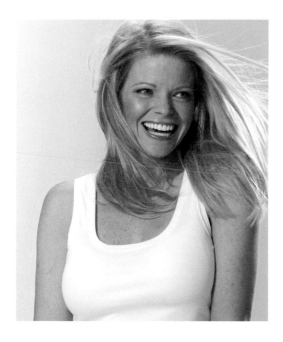

My longtime best friend,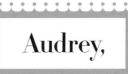

Audrey,

and I met when we were both twelve. Well, she was almost thirteen—seven months older than me. That is our running joke. Boy, do I milk being a year younger than she is by those seven months.

Audrey started coming to my school in New Baltimore, Michigan, when she and her family moved into a house down the street from me. She was this beautiful girl who really didn't seem to be bothered by what anyone else at school was up to. She always seemed to be busy and have somewhere to go, almost like there was no one else in the school but her.

I was intrigued. Who was this girl? ("Girl" would later become one of the many nicknames I gave her over the years.) I had to figure her out. This came in the form of me, a screaming 12-year-old boy, doing donuts on her front lawn on my snowmobile, yelling, "HEY, NEW GIRL! HEY, NEW GIRL!" (Did I already mention how shy I was?)

Somehow we became best friends. And yes, I was actually very shy. Audrey has always had an amazing air of confidence about her. This is one of the many things I love about her. If I was being shy or hesitant, she would say, "Oh, Kenney, come on…" We were like the junior-high version of Bonnie and Clyde. With my best friend Audrey by my side, I really opened up. All we needed was each other.

Audrey is an amazing woman. She is kind, thoughtful, and supportive. She went through school and college with good grades, graduating as a registered nurse. Audrey is now the amazing mother of four boys, including my godson Zach. I am happy to say, she is just as nutty with her kids as we were when we were young—although sometimes I feel her kids are more mature than we are now!

"Carol," as I like to call her, juggles it all. Audrey recently attended a beauty-editor event in New York as a model for me. I had to announce to all the editors that Audrey was sorry, but she had to leave early to catch a flight back to South Carolina in time to stop off at Ingles (her local grocery store) to pick up dinner for her husband and kids—all while sporting a perfect ponytail and freshly applied lip-gloss! True story. I love that about her!

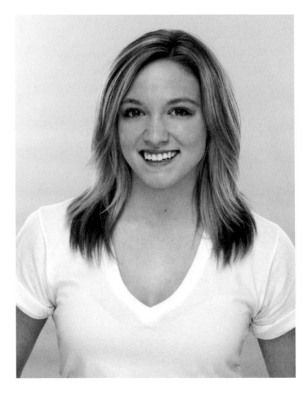

My niece 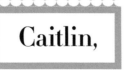 or Cakee Doodle, as I like to call her, has always been my little princess. She is a beautiful girl. As a child, she had the biggest, most beautiful blue eyes and the blondest of blonde hair. She was such a little doll. Caitlin also grew up to be quite competitive and fierce on the soccer field and in other sports.

I have definitely bought Caitlin her share of high heels, dresses, makeup, and hair extensions, and I've included Caitlin as a model for many of the projects I've worked on. What I admire the most about Caitlin is that she is in *no way* defined by the way she looks. If anything, this is an afterthought for Caitlin, who defines herself by her capabilities (she's smart, talented, athletic, creative, resourceful, good in school, friendly) and how she treats other people. Caitlin is not afraid to work hard for what she wants. I also remember taking her shopping, and she'd say to me, "That's OK, Uncle Kenney, I don't need a new jacket, you already bought me something similar." What teenage girl says that? Caitlin.

Caitlin has always been considerate of others. She has visited homeless shelters with me, delivered Christmas gifts to children who are less fortunate, taken Thanksgiving dinner to people who are homeless, helped me raise money for charity, and visited Honduras, at age 13, on a mission with me and Operation Smile to help children who were undergoing cleft-lip and cleft-palate surgery. I can honestly say I am so proud of the young woman Caitlin has become. She is kind, considerate, loving, determined, dedicated, compassionate—and beautiful. Love you, Cakes!

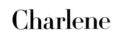

Charlene is my good friend, but we also call each other brother and sister. She is an accomplished woman with a great career as a successful celebrity clothing stylist and lifestyle brand designer, and she did it all on her own. Charlene is bubbly and funny but also chic as can be. She has a heart of gold and royal taste. Charlene and I started off in the business together and have known each other for many years. I have seen firsthand how hard she has worked on her own to get where she is today. Despite the hard work, she has always made time to be a great friend. We have worked and traveled the world together, often sharing the same room. We laugh hard together and love what we do. Charlene comes from humble begin- nings, as do I, and she is no stranger to giving back.

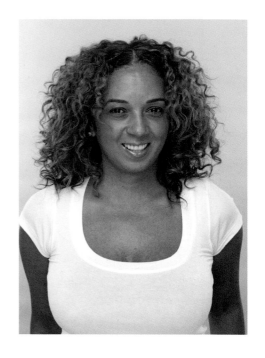

I knew I could count on Charlene when Leeza Gibbons asked me to be one of the hosts of an Oscar event with her and David Foster that was taking place at Mr. Chow, a famous eatery in Beverly Hills. Leeza's goal was to give the event a heart and purpose. Each of us would bring the values we cared for most to the event. I wanted to make a point that we need to stop taking each other at face value, and I decided to work with a group of homeless women from a shelter Leeza supported. Since the women were all trying to get into the workforce, I wanted to help prepare them with a makeover, but I also wanted to celebrate them on the red carpet at an Oscar event. Charlene and I made over each of the women. Charlene treated them with great dignity and respect, as she would any of her celebrity clients. She dressed them in gowns and covered them in jewels. For the first time these women stood on the other side of the velvet rope, with the world (and the paparazzi) watching and wondering who they were.

I didn't tell anyone the women's story. We didn't want them to be judged the way that people usually saw them. It was an empowering moment, at the end of the event, when one of the women told her story on a live broadcast. Not many people would have worked as hard to honor these women as Charlene did, especially during Oscar week, one of the busiest times for us in Los Angeles. She gave them her all. That is Charlene, a stylish heart of gold.

My sister-in-law, **Lisa,** is married to my brother Jon, and the mother of Caitlin, Ethan, and Chloe. Lisa is also my guardian angel Ryan's mother. (Please see page 248 for more about Ryan.) I have known Lisa since I was nine years old and noticed that we both wore our hair in the same feathered hairstyle. Lisa and my brother Jon were high-school sweethearts. They started dating in the ninth grade and married after high school. I always tell Jon that if I wasn't me, the next person I would want to be is him. I have always admired Jon and Lisa for their relationship and their family (they're wonderful parents). Lisa is an amazing and beautiful woman and a great role model for her children.

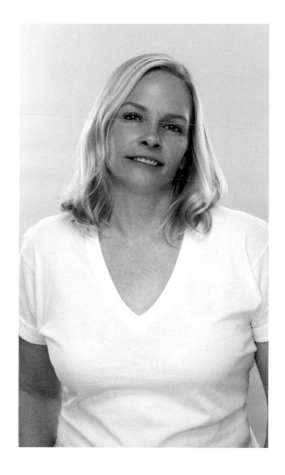

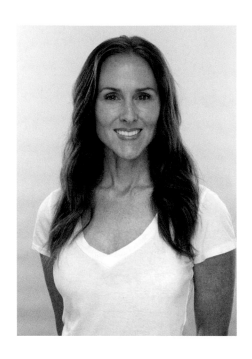

Sarah

Siegel Magness is like a sister to me, and one of the most caring, consistent, and driven women I know. She and her husband financed and produced the Oscar-nominated film *Precious*, and she is an accomplished director, entrepreneur, wife, mother, and friend. I say consistent because most people change when they are in different environments or situations, but Sarah is such a confident woman that she is always Sarah—the same amazingly levelheaded, compassionate person, no matter what. I always call her for advice, especially when I am afraid that I am acting irrationally!

My longtime friend, 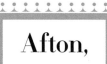 ## Afton, is like a spiritual mother to me. I call her Mother Afton. She is all love and positive energy. Afton calms and envelops you. Afton follows her soul and encourages me to think beyond my brain, with my whole body and spirit. She has taught me to breathe, meditate, and find inner peace. Afton is also the woman who gave me my four lovely children—my Salukis—including Afton, my oldest, who is named after her, and my other dogs, Taj, Honoree, and Jedah.

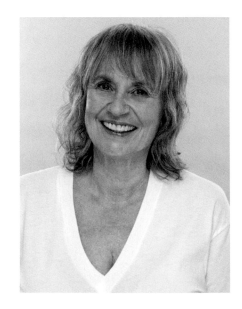

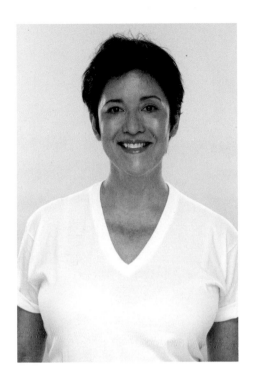

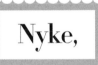

Chloe is my dear friend and creative director of the Ken Paves Salon Los Angeles. Chloe inspires me not only as an artist, but as a human being, too. Chloe and I also share a very spiritual connection. We are believers in fate: Everything happens for a reason. Chloe is also an amazing wife and mother. I have watched her work very hard and never compromise raising her son, Alec. After school, while she was working, Alec would do his homework in the garden at the salon. Chloe would arrange her schedule to be there for all his important moments. She loves life and everyone in it.

When I met **Nyke,** (Nyeisha) Prince, my friend and assistant, she was a budding hairstylist as well as a drummer and model between jobs. I happened to be looking for an assistant who could travel with me full-time. Nyke fit the job description perfectly.

Nyke and I also have something else in common: We both speak American sign language. Nyke is deaf, and I went to college to work with deaf children before going to beauty school. It was a match made in hair heaven. Nyke and I have traveled the world together and become great friends.

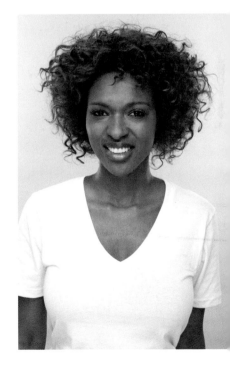

Lesli

and I have known each other for twelve years. She was a powerhouse attorney for many of my celeb clients. Before I actually met her, I'd hear about a lawyer named Lesli, whom some called "The Cleaner." I imagined that Lesli would be a burly Scottish guy…Nope. Lesli's all California blonde—beach native Lesli!

Lesli became my lawyer years ago, although I didn't need anything cleaned, and she is now my manager as well. Lesli has an incredible work ethic and is the mother of two great kids, Blair and Jake.

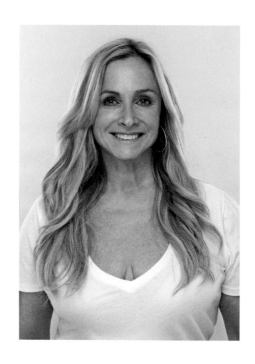

Blair

is Lesli's mother. OK, she's not really her mom, but she often acts like the mother in certain situations.

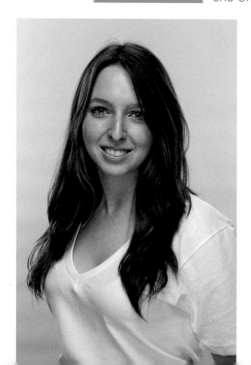

If Lesli is a minute past her "curfew," she'll be greeted by Blair, with her arms crossed, outside the front door of their house. Blair usually says something like this: "I hope you're happy you're late. I was worried and didn't know what to do, so I cleaned the kitchen, did the dishes, and made your bed. Get in here! Where were you?!"

Blair is truly a beautiful young woman who is going to college now. She finished high school at a magnet program associated with the Los Angeles Zoo—so that she can work with big animals one day.

We always joke that Blair is my adopted daughter. We spent a lot of time together when she was growing up. Blair fascinates me and, ever since I can remember, she has always had her own thoughts about things. Not only is Blair a beautiful and intellectual young woman, with an amazing head of hair, she also exudes a sense of confidence and self-worth that is never compromised by anyone else or their standards.

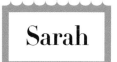

Sarah Lucero and I met just a few years ago, when we were working together with Victoria Beckham (we still do). She is a talented makeup artist and the global creative director for Stila cosmetics. I remember being in awe of her nearly waist-length, gorgeous, extension-free, natural dirty blonde hair! She had the perfect beach hair that I was always trying to give to other people—she just woke up like that. I have gotten to know Sarah as a kind and lovely woman. She is gentle and considerate. One day Victoria called me and asked if I would do her a favor. She said that Sarah had just been diagnosed with breast cancer and would lose her hair from chemotherapy treatments. She asked if I would make Sarah a wig before all her hair fell out. With the help of one of the stylists at my salon, Alexis Kuykendall,

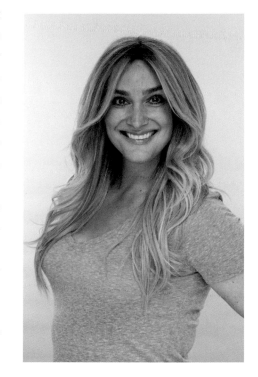

I made a wig as close to Sarah's natural hair as I could. I am proud and honored that Sarah will share her story later in these pages. Now a cancer survivor, Sarah has become an advocate for other women who are going through cancer.

· · · · · · · · · · · ·

As you see, all the ladies look great. At the photo shoot, it made me proud to see them, these women who are so important to me, sitting together and looking so beautiful—just as themselves.

Taking those first pictures, though, was an adventure for some of the women. Their reactions, understandably, were mixed:

"I was excited to come!" said Caitlin. "But I was also a little nervous because you're put on the spot when you're in front of the camera. It's not something you do every day. You have all these eyes on you and people saying, 'Stand like this! Turn like this! Act natural!' You feel like— 'Is this a fake smile? A real smile? I don't know what I'm doing right now!' It's nerve-wracking when you don't know what you look like in the picture!"

Tip and Lisa said they were excited about the shoot. "This is so outside my normal life," said Lisa, who came to the shoot from Michigan. "I'm looking forward to maybe going home with some new ideas—quick things I can do to make things easier and look more put together."

At the other end of the spectrum was Audrey, who said, "The no makeup part is not happening. I put lip liner and bronzer on before I even open the door for the UPS man. Kenney doesn't even go out without a tan. Who's he kidding?"

While my mom, Helen, said she was happy to be there, she added, "I feel uncomfortable having people watch me while I'm being photo-graphed." Looking at Afton, she said, "It is very intimidating."

Afton agreed. "I've never done anything like this. I feel intimidated! But Ken said, 'Come to the shoot just the way you come to my house.' I felt much better."

Sarah M. said she doesn't mind having her picture taken, "but only if they look good!" she laughed. "If you smile it's always a good picture."

During the shoot, and throughout this book, I've asked each of these amazing women to share their experiences and thoughts about beauty and how it plays out in real life.

What *real women* have to say about...

When They Feel Most Beautiful

Helen: *"Sitting outside, reading a book. A nice conversation with my family or a good friend. Doing something for myself or someone else. The love of my family. I feel most beautiful being me. I've lived a good life and feel like I did my best to be a good person, a good wife, a good mother, and the best Helen I could be."*

Lisa: *"Taking time to do something for myself. As a mother of three children who are involved in many different activities, I rarely take time for me and put everyone else's needs first. When I actually take the time to do something for myself, such as going to the gym to lift weights and run on the treadmill, I feel better about myself and therefore take more care when I'm doing my hair and makeup and getting dressed. All of this creates a happier mom who has more energy and is a lot more fun to be around."*

Chloe: *"I feel most beautiful when I am living in the present moment—when I can see myself, flaws and all, and just accept myself as is. This is when I remind myself that I am the only Chloe in this whole universe. Nobody can take that from me!"*

Caitlin: *"I feel most beautiful when I get my hair to cooperate with a minimal amount of work and wear very light makeup. I don't prefer to be overly made up, not on a daily basis, at least. I feel that less truly is more, and I feel most comfortable in my own skin that way."*

Audrey: *"I feel the most beautiful and the proudest when I look at my kids. I have four boys. Cory, who is nineteen, is a freshman in college. Anthony, fourteen, is a freshman in high school. Ken's godson, Zach, is eleven. My youngest, Joey, is nine. I want to be the best wife I can be to my husband, and the most amazing mom I can be to my sons. It's so important to me to raise them to be good men and to do well in life. When I watched my son get a football award last year—it was his first season playing tackle football—I felt beautiful because I had raised this child and was so proud of him."*

Nyke: *"I feel the most beautiful when I'm in the dance studio. I feel beautiful in my ballet outfits and when I dance in front of the big mirror in the studio. That's when people get to see the real me."*

Afton: *"I feel beautiful when I dress for myself. How dressed up or down I am makes no difference. Actually, when I take the most trouble to get ready for something, I feel least myself. I feel good when I'm managing my diet and exercise, and of course, feedback from others gives me confidence that makes me radiate beauty."*

Sarah M: *"I feel the most beautiful when I'm happy and with my family. Beauty comes from within. If we feel good inside, beauty radiates on the outside. Happy people are always the most beautiful…*

Beauty is in our attitude, philosophy, and outlook on the future. The best beauty regimen I have is to wake up, state out loud why I am grateful, set good intentions for the day, and listen to music that gets me energized to make the best of my day."

Tip: *"I always feel beautiful. I have a healthy body and a great life and I'm happy. There's nothing to bring me down, really. I like who I am. I like that I'm positive and sunny and never negative. I feel like I'm a good friend and support people wherever I can."*

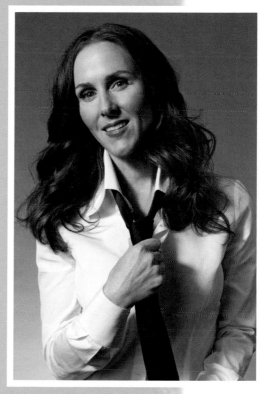

Sarah M. looking fabulous!

Charlene: *"Life makes me feel beautiful. So does happiness, great health, and close friends. It's not about how I feel on the outside—it's what gives me joy on the inside that makes me glow! I start my day reading the Bible. I take time out to pray in the morning. That keeps me flowing throughout the day."*

Lesli: *"I feel the most beautiful when I relax and live in the moment."*

Blair: *"I feel the most beautiful when I get compliments about what I'm wearing or what I've done with my hair—especially when I get them from Ken because I know he has worked with so many beautiful girls and women. So when he says, 'Wow, Blair, you look beautiful,' those are the times when I feel unstoppable."*

Sarah L: *"I feel the most beautiful when I take time to appreciate all the beauty around me—nature, the sun—and time spent with loved ones and friends. Smiling and laughing make me feel beautiful. I think when you feel comfortable—that is beautiful.*

Just for fun, *I asked my friend, famed photographer Richard Mclaren, who took all the gorgeous shots in this book, when he feels the most beautiful. Richard, who kept the shoot lively with his quick wit, made us all laugh again when he said in his thick English accent, "I was born beautiful!"*

Feeling beautiful comes down to accepting and loving who you are and what you look like right now. You might look in the mirror and say, "Is this it?" Yes, that's it! Even if it's what you might not want, you must accept yourself in this moment and recognize the beauty staring back at you.

Over the years, I've found that so many women want what they don't have. Women with fine, straight hair want big, bouncy curls. Woman with curly hair want to smooth theirs out. This is the moment to say, "You know what? This is me, this is what I have, and I love what I have." Don't stop saying this until you truly believe it. Once you believe it, together we can start enhancing it.

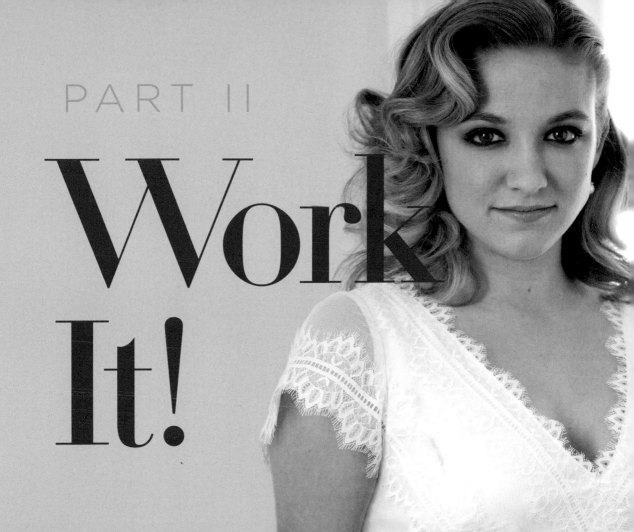

PART II

Work It!

"I don't like myself,

I'm crazy about myself."

—MAE WEST

Now that you know how much you have to work with, I will offer some tips in this section to help you to have the best hair imaginable and to look and feel your best, every single day.

GETTING DOWN
to the Roots

I hope you realize—or have started to realize—what a beautiful woman you are inside and out, by accepting who you are and what you look like at this very moment.

Fully accepting who you are, though, isn't always easy.

The solution lies in learning how to take care of yourself in all aspects of your life, so you feel better about who you are and what you look like. It all goes back to self-love. When you treat yourself well by taking time to care for your body, hair, skin, and nails, and when you nourish your soul by doing things you like and surrounding yourself with upbeat people and positive experiences, your whole outlook brightens. Give yourself the attention you deserve. Life is good because you feel good, on the inside and out, even if you have chunky thighs, a few wrinkles around your eyes, or hair with a mind of its own.

Here's some tough love. We're not getting any younger, so, as my good friend Ellen Rakieten says, "Don't waste the pretty!"

If you can't accept yourself now, what are you going to do next year? I'll tell you what. You'll wish you could go back to this year. So live now, embrace life, and "don't waste the pretty!"

I'm going to give you some tips to change things that you might want to improve, *for you*—not because you feel pressured to look or act like someone you're not or because someone made a comment about something you did or the way you look, but because you want to make the most of what you've got, and feel the best you can, physically and mentally, right now.

You don't have to follow all the tips in this book. Try one or two at first. Take things slowly, if that's what makes you comfortable. You're in the driver's seat here. It's your life. Do what you want to do. You might read something here and say, "No way, Ken!" But then, after you let things percolate a while or see how one tip improved something that's been bugging you, you might change your mind and say, "OK, maybe I'll try that other thing. Let's see what happens." It's all about treating yourself with TLC.

So many women tell me what a lift they get when they're having a great hair day. When your hair looks good, you feel good. So in this chapter I will suggest how to care for your hair in the best way possible, with simple solutions that don't require a lot of time or money, but will leave your hair looking healthier and you feeling more confident.

It's Your Hair ... Accept It

One of the biggest problems I have with the beauty industry today is that it preys on women's insecurities and causes them to be overly critical of themselves. The real motivating force behind the industry is to get you to spend a fortune on beauty products—the assumption being that you have something (a lot!) that needs to be fixed. I'm here to tell you that you don't.

In this chapter, I want you to recognize your hair type and not only accept it, but learn to love it. If you have fine, straight hair, work with it; if you have tight curls, you don't have to straighten them; if your hair is curly underneath, wavy in the middle, and somewhat straight on top, that's fine too—learn to love it!

Do you have tight, kinky curls or coarse hair? Is your hair wavy, fine, stick-straight, or limp? Does your hair get oily a few hours after washing it? Is it as dry as the Mohave Desert? Or is it some of both—oily in some spots and dry in others? Knowing what kind of hair texture and type you have will help you to take care of it the way you should.

Although the four different hair types are curly, straight, wavy, and kinky—and the three types of hair textures are coarse, medium, and fine—keep in mind that your hair can be a combination of these textures and types. All I want you to do is to understand your hair. So once you know your type and texture, please say it out loud and proud!

> *"I have five wavy hairs that I try to make look like seven."*
>
> —CHERI OTERI,
> *actress & comedienne*

It's Your Crowning Glory— Let's Make It Shine

When you get the basics down and do all the right things for your hair, your tresses will look and act the way you want—shiny, sexy, gorgeous, and manageable. I guarantee that when you feel good about your hair, you will feel better about yourself.

When I'm working with clients or makeover candidates, I always stress how important it is to have healthy hair. The key to turning everyday hair into glamorous, luxurious hair is to get it into the best condition possible. It's just that simple. Your hair is a reflection of your health. Just as you want a fit body, luminous skin, and strong nails, you want your hair to be as healthy as possible to look and feel your best.

The Right Shampoo

Using a sulfate-free shampoo is the first step to getting and keeping your hair healthy, shiny, and soft. Stay away from hair products that contain sodium laureth sulfate or sodium lauryl ether sulfate (SLES), which is the main ingredient in dish detergent, believe it or not. SLES strips oil off

A little goes a long way.

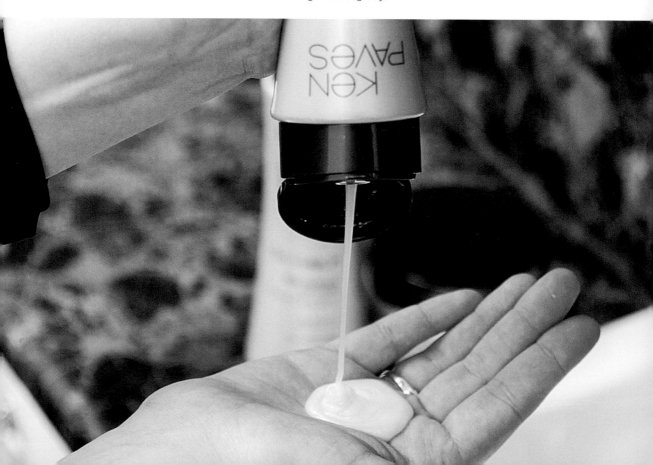

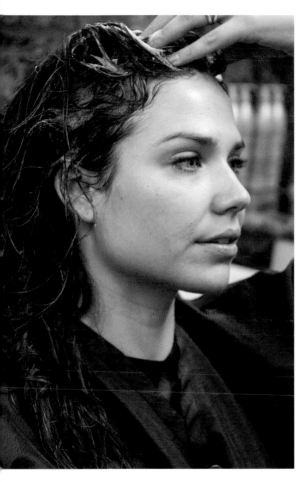

Lather just the roots of your hair.

dishes. So it's definitely going to strip the natural oils—your greatest defense against damage—from your hair and scalp. There's no better conditioner than your own natural oils.

If you love the feeling of a rich lather when you're washing your hair, you don't have to give that up. It's easy to find sulfate-free shampoos that lather nicely and feel rich and luxurious. Just check the label first before you buy the product.

Shampooing Savvy

Hair is usually very healthy at the root, but the midshaft and ends tend to get dry and brittle. This is because only your roots are benefiting from the natural oils that you keep stripping from your hair by overcleansing.

If you're like most women, you scrub all your hair with shampoo when you get into the shower. Every strand. This is a shampooing *don't*. Lather only the roots, where hair produces the most oil. Shampooing the ends of your hair will only dry them out. Don't worry—they'll still get clean without scrubbing.

Resist the urge to pile all your hair on top of your head when shampooing. There's no need to do this. Instead, tip your head over in the shower, put some shampoo on the top of your head and massage your entire scalp, especially around the hairline and the back of the head, where the roots of your hair meet the nape of your neck. These are the areas that tend to get the oiliest. When you rinse, some residual shampoo will reach the ends. This is far less harmful than mushing your hair on top of your head and rubbing shampoo all over it.

Another trick is to wet your hair and let it fall to your shoulders, shampooing only the first inch or two of hair from your scalp down. Focus again on massaging the whole scalp with your fingers, not the palm of your hands. That's what I like to do when I'm washing my own hair as well as my clients'.

Even though the directions on shampoo bottles often say, "Lather, rinse, and repeat," this does not apply to everyone. (Shampoo manufacturers just want you to use more of their product—and use it up faster—so that you'll have to buy more.) For most people, once is usually enough.

One other thing, ladies—remember how I told you to be gentle when it comes to your hair? *Never, ever wash* your hair with scalding hot water. Caring for the cuticle, the outermost layer of the hair, is key. The cuticle seals and protects your hair, keeping in the natural oils and hair-dye molecules as well. Washing your hair with

> SOMETIMES WHEN I TELL WOMEN to shampoo only their roots, they say, "Wait just one minute. That sounds strange." While reading some of these tips, you may stop and think, "This doesn't make much sense. It seems so simple." But after a month of shampooing your hair the right way and following a few more hair-care tips, you will definitely notice a huge difference in your hair. You'll also feel better about yourself because you took charge.

superhot water will dry out not only your hair, but your skin, too, particularly in the winter months. Washing your hair with cooler water, on the other hand, helps maintain the health of your hair as well as the longevity of your hair color, if you dye your hair. If you can bear it, finish your shower with a blast of cold water—which helps close the cuticles and makes your hair shinier. (Cold water also boosts circulation in your entire body—and will wake you up!)

How Often to Suds Up

Avoid shampooing your hair every day. For very dry and coarse hair, once a week may be often enough. Otherwise, washing your hair two to three times a week is sufficient. Some women say they have to shower and wash their hair every day. Keep in mind, however, that water alone is responsible for eroding mountains, so it can certainly do a good job of dissolving your natural oils.

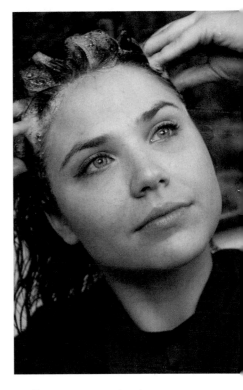

If you feel the need for "freshly washed" hair every day, try this instead: rinse your hair thoroughly with warm water, concentrating on and massaging your roots. Then condition your hair, from the midshaft to the ends (or just the areas that feel dry). The water will give you the clean (but not stripped) feeling that you desire, and the conditioner will leave your hair soft and smelling fresh.

You can also try a dry shampoo between washes to soak up excess oil and pump up the volume of your hair a bit.

Focus on your roots whenever you suds up.

Conditioning 101

Conditioner is supposed to mimic what your natural oils are intended to do—hydrate, protect, nourish, and improve the condition of your hair. At one time, women were encouraged to brush their hair one hundred times a night, the idea being that brushing would help natural oils travel the length of the hair and condition it. That may have worked, my friend, until women really started abusing their hair. Now they need all the help they can get to repair it, which is where the many forms of conditioner come in.

Washing, drying, coloring, styling—plus countless environmental aggressors—all dry out your hair. Natural oils can't possibly keep up. The texture of your hair also plays a role in how easily it becomes dehydrated. Each hair grows from a single follicle in the scalp. At the base of

Cosmetic chemist Alec Batis of Batis Marketing Concept, Inc., on conditioning

When you have healthy hair that has never been colored, permed, or highlighted, nothing can get inside the hair shaft because it's still got its guts—it's resilient. But when you chemically treat your hair by highlighting or bleaching it, for instance, you hollow out the hair shaft, damaging and drying it. Conditioners with heavy silicones make your hair look healthy for a while but hide the fact that it's still damaged and dry. Silicones are not treatment ingredients. They simply smooth the hair shaft, giving the illusion of health, shine, and manageability. There is nothing wrong with this. Think of it as makeup for your hair—like using a bronzer to give you the appearance of youth and radiance.

Thankfully there are many types of silicones. Be sure to pick light silicones that have a weightless conditioning effect—especially the follicle is the papilla, the bulb of the hair where most growth takes place. Right where the hair grows out of your scalp, there is a sebaceous oil gland, which nourishes your hair beneath the scalp, the scalp itself, and the base of the hair shaft. However, the hair that has grown out of your scalp is no longer living; it is, basically, a dead fiber. Therefore, you need a conditioner to keep it soft, supple, shiny, and manageable.

Conditioning your hair is one of the most important things you can do to take care of it. The goal of conditioning is to make the cuticle, that outermost layer of your hair, lie flat and smooth. The cuticle is made up of layers that resemble fish scales. These scales either rise open or seal shut. When the fibers of the cuticle are raised or open, hair is vulnerable, making it look dull, dry, and brittle. When the cuticle is closed, it acts as a protective shield and helps to seal in moisture. A

if you have damaged or chemically treated hair. Think of it this way: While heavy, matte makeup looks caked on, sheer, light makeup makes your skin look fresh and healthy. It's the same with your hair. You want to look for conditioners that contain weightless silicones such as dimethicone and phenyl dimethicone.

You also want to nourish your hair by eating plenty of fruits, vegetables, and omega-3-rich foods, such as salmon, nuts, and seeds, and by using products that contain nourishing ingredients such as Co-Q10, as well as lipids, emollients, and essential oils, such as omega-3 (linolenic acid) and omega-6, coconut oil, olive oil, tamanu oil, and argan oil. Be wary of products that contain lipids that are very far down the ingredient list. This means there's not much of that ingredient in the formula. Lipids and emollients work at the root level to draw in moisture to the skin cells in the scalp, strengthening the follicle to grow strong healthy hair.

cuticle that lies flat also results in smooth, manageable, shiny hair. Also, when the cuticle is flat it becomes reflective and appears shiny, like any other smooth surface. Although curly hair has a natural tendency to have a more raised cuticle, all hair types benefit from a smooth cuticle.

Conditioning the Cuticle

So, ladies, after Hair Conditioning 101, let's condition your cuticles. Keep in mind, however, that all hair is much weaker when it is wet, so handle it with care.

Now that you know the importance of conditioning, you need to figure out where you need it. Just as we discussed with shampooing, it is important to condition your hair only where it needs it for routine conditioning. Most people's hair is healthy at the root and would benefit from being conditioned starting one to two inches from the scalp all

The Wonders of Olive Oil

You don't have to invest in expensive products to keep your hair hydrated and healthy. I love using olive oil on dry, coarse, curly, or processed hair because it is made up of tiny molecules that are similar to the molecules in your hair's natural oils. These molecules penetrate your cuticles more easily than some store-bought conditioning agents, which have larger molecules—and which also condition your hair well, but do so by sitting on top of your hair.

I like to put olive oil in a non-aerosol atomizer, the kind you use in your kitchen to mist oil onto food and cookware. I mix about 30 percent olive oil with 70 percent water, shake it, and spray it on the ends of hair, from the midshaft down, section by section. (You can also pour the mixture onto your hair.) Do not apply oil to your roots because they don't need any extra oil.

the way to the ends of the hair. However, very fine, limp hair may be healthy a few inches out from the scalp and may only need to be conditioned from the midshaft to the ends. By conditioning your hair only where you need it, you'll avoid an oily scalp and limp hair. Very short hair doesn't normally get weighed down the same way as long hair; use only as much conditioner as you truly need and rinse thoroughly.

There are, of course, exceptions. Very coarse hair or hair that

SOMETIMES WHEN I'M TRAVELING with a client who has a TV interview or photo shoot the next day, the first thing I do when we get to the hotel (especially after a long flight) is ask room service to send up a small bowl of olive oil. (I always wonder what they think I'm going to do with it!) I spray the olive oil and water mixture onto my client's hair and leave it on overnight. The next morning, after washing, conditioning, and styling, her hair looks lustrous and rich. Instant glamour!

I recommend leaving the oil and water mixture on your hair for a couple of hours or overnight while you sleep. (If you leave the mixture on your hair overnight, wrap your hair in a scarf to avoid getting oil on your skin or pillowcase.) If you don't usually wash your hair in the morning, you can spray the olive oil mixture on your ends and leave it on for a few hours—the more time, the better. Or, if you're just going to be hanging around the house, you can don a shower cap to lock in the heat from your head. You can even try a

heating cap, like my friend, Charlene, uses. Then wash, condition, and style your hair as usual. The olive oil will leave your hair hydrated, silkier looking, and baby soft. It won't leave your ends greasy at all. You can do this once a month, or more often, depending on your hair's texture and how dry it is.

is dry due to excessive chemical processing may require routine root-to-end conditioning. Also monthly or deep conditioning treatments are often done from the roots to the ends.

Always choose a conditioner that contains essential oils that are beneficial to the hair as a natural hydrator.

Finding the Right Conditioner

Using the right conditioner will go a long way toward getting and keeping your hair its healthiest. Keep in mind that a lot of conditioners contain heavy silicones, which coat your cuticles with an artificial barrier. It's like slathering your hair with floor wax.

When you start using conditioners that contain heavier silicone,

Chamomile Tea Is Not Just for Drinking

Chamomile tea is another at-home remedy I tell my clients to use. It's a natural toner that gives hair a warm honey hue. It will also add depth to faded, dull blonde hair.

To treat your hair with chamomile tea, boil some water, drop in a teabag, and let it steep. After the tea cools, wash your hair, condition it, pour the tea over your hair, and let it dry. This will give your color a boost and a healthy glow, but not permanently—it will only last until your next shampoo. You can use darker-colored teas for darker hair. For example, strong black tea will tone black hair, while hibiscus tea, paprika, or rosehips enhance reddish tones.

your hair feels great for a while. After rinsing it off wet hair, it feels slippery, so you think it's working. You use the conditioner religiously, thinking you're doing something good for your hair. But then, maybe six to eight months later, you may come to find that your hair seems weighed down, drier than ever, dull, and lifeless.

Deep Conditioning

If you have dry, coarse, curly, processed, or badly damaged hair, I recommend using a deep conditioner or a hot oil treatment at least once a week, or twice a month for less-damaged hair, to keep it well moisturized.

When you use a deep conditioner in the shower, throw on a shower cap to trap the heat from the warm water. This will open up the cuticles and let the conditioner seep deeper into the hair shaft.

Deep Conditioning Boosters

There are many amazing deep conditioners on the market that will give tired, overworked tresses a moisture boost. But you can also use natural ingredients that you already have at home and that will hydrate your hair just as well. I whipped up these deep conditioning boosters with the team from *The Doctors* for a segment that aired in 2011:

• For dry, curly, coarse, or kinky hair, I like to use a banana mask that hydrates hair really well. All you have to do is whip 1 tablespoon of olive oil, 1 egg, and ½ banana in a bowl, then apply it to your hair using your hands or a tint brush, section by section, from the midshaft to the ends. Leave the mixture on your hair for twenty minutes or so, preferably underneath a shower cap. Then wash, condition, and style your hair as usual—it will look shinier than it has in a long time.

• If you have fine or oily hair, you want to soak up as much oil on the roots as possible without drying the ends. I like to use essential

continued on the next page

Deep Conditioning Boosters continued

oils, which are amazing for hair and skin. While you want to avoid greasy-looking hair, you still want to get the benefits of natural oils. To accomplish this, I make a mixture of apple cider vinegar, which removes any buildup of excess oils on the hair, and some emollients to gently hydrate the hair. I like to use a drop or two of mandarin orange or lavender essential oil with a squeeze of fresh lemon to help the hair rinse clear.

Put this mixture into a non-aerosol atomizer, shake it, and then spray it onto the hair from the root to the midshaft. (You can also pour the mixture on with a cup or bowl.) Don't spray the mixture on the ends, since they don't need it.

Leave the mixture on your hair for about twenty minutes to blot up excess oils. Then wash, condition, and style your hair as usual. It will look shiny and feel soft—without a greasy feel. You can do this once a week or twice a month, depending on the texture and oiliness of your hair.

What *real women* have to say about...

Conditioning

"I've been really into my hair since I was a little girl," says Charlene. *Every one or two weeks I put a mask on my hair with a heating cap. I use Amla oil from India. I also put a mixture of olive oil and hemp oil on my scalp. My curly hair gets so dry because the oils from my scalp don't get to the ends. So every night—religiously—I use an oil treatment. I apply it to my hair and then wash it out the next day (or sometimes the day after). I take vitamins for my hair, too, to promote healthy growth."*

Hair Drying 101

Now, some of you may shudder when you read this, but my best advice for healthy hair is to let it air-dry. I know, I know. I hear it all the time from my clients: "Ken! My hair looks like a rat's nest if I don't blow-dry it straight and flat iron or curl it every day!"

Here's the deal. Your hair is the most fragile when it is wet. Hair can absorb 30 percent of its weight in water. Porous or coarse hair can absorb up to 50 percent of its weight in water. Remember how important the cuticle layer of the hair is—hair is its strongest when the cuticle is lying flat, acting as a protective shield. When hair is wet, the cuticle is not lying flat. Instead, the cuticle expands, leaving the interior of the hair compromised. When hair is wet, it is swollen. To add insult to injury, you weaken and even break swollen strands of hair by stretching them with a brush while applying heat as you blow-dry. Imagine drinking two gallons of water, then immediately doing intense yoga in a 105-degree room. That's what you're doing to your hair every time you blow-dry it when it's wet.

This is why I prefer air-drying. I recommend applying a hydrating hair serum to towel-dried hair and then allowing it to air-dry completely. The serum, applied to dry areas of your hair, will help maintain the moisture it needs while it dries. The serum also encourages the cuticle to lie flat and helps make it strong and protective while acting as a barrier against heat styling. Believe it or not, your hair is more resilient to heat-styling damage if it is already dry. Try it! Let your hair air-dry or work off second-day hair and touch it up, either with a flat iron, curling iron, or hot rollers.

Some hair may also air-dry beautifully and not need any additional styling. Again, this is why I want you to embrace and love your texture.

If you shower every day, try not to get your hair wet each time and just touch it up between shampoos.

I am not saying to never blow-dry your hair. I am just saying to take it easy and give your hair a rest. Save the full blow-dry for once a week or for a special occasion. You will soon notice a difference in the condition of your hair.

Hair-Drying Tips

Here are a few ways to gently dry your hair without damaging it:

♦ After shampooing and conditioning, towel-dry your hair by squeezing it gently with the towel, not roughing it up. Remember, a wet cuticle is raised and will snag other cuticles like barbed wire, causing knots and snarls.

♦ Apply serum or detangler to your hands and then run it through your hair where it needs it the most. Concentrate on the ends, since this will help seal any split ends. As you run product through your hair with your hands, remember to go section by section, and don't forget the underneath and inside sections of your hair.

♦ Most women mistakenly run product just over the top of their hair. Once your hair is towel-dried and you've applied either a serum or leave-in conditioner, your cuticle should be lying flat, and you can now use a wide-tooth comb to detangle your hair.

♦ You can also add a styling product to achieve your desired look, whether it is volume or sleekness you're after. Volumizing products tend to open and expand the cuticle, increasing the diameter of each hair strand, so concentrate on using these products from the root to the midshaft, where volume is needed, and leave the ends hydrated with the serum or detangler. For a smooth, sleek look, I apply the smoothing product from roots to end.

◆ In order to maximize the benefits of any hair product, you must also distribute the product into the interior sections of your hair, not just on top. Now that your hair is prepped, this is a great time to let your hair air-dry.

◆ Keep in mind that wet hair tends to frizz even more when you play with it with your hands. The wet and expanded cuticle layer of the hair catches on the raised ridges on your fingertips and lifts the cuticle even more.

How to Blow-Dry Your Hair the Right Way

Back to blow-drying, which I've been avoiding, trying to get you to avoid it. But if you must, try these tips:

◆ To start, I recommend drying your hair with your fingers. This not only helps eliminate moisture, while reducing damage to your hair from too much heat and overdrying, but also reduces blow-dry and styling time.

◆ Keeping your dryer a safe distance from your hair (four to six inches away), begin drying it in the back, with your hair parted down the middle. Tilt your head forward and direct the air down the length of your hair, in the same direction as the cuticle—which runs downward from the scalp toward the end of each hair—while smoothing your hair with your fingers. This will help close the cuticle. Never dry your hair going against the direction of the cuticle.

- Most people really fry the top of their hair (the crown), because they blow-dry this area with hot air focused right on top—where the hair continues to get heated long after it is dry. (This is why you need to begin drying sections of your hair from the back.)

- Before you begin using a brush, continue to finger-dry sections of your hair, working forward from the back of your head until your hair is about 70 percent dry. This will eliminate enough moisture to strengthen the hair but still leave in enough moisture to keep it elastic, so that you can gently stretch it into whatever shape you desire.

- Once the back sections of your hair are 70 percent dry, begin blow-drying the top and sides of your hair (with your hair parted). Make sure to tilt your head to the side and direct the blow drier downward, under your hair along the side sections, so that you don't dry the crown of your hair too much. As you did with the back sections, continue to blow-dry side sections until they're about 70 percent dry. If the styling product you're using has been well distributed, you may be amazed at how well your hair texture is already turning out.

- Finish blow-drying your hair from the back and repeat the pattern (of drying your hair in sections) using a flat or round brush, depending on the result you want. Thick, coarse hair may require blow-drying in small sections to achieve the desired look. If possible, clip sections away as you work from the back of your head to the front.

Blow-drying Caitlin's hair

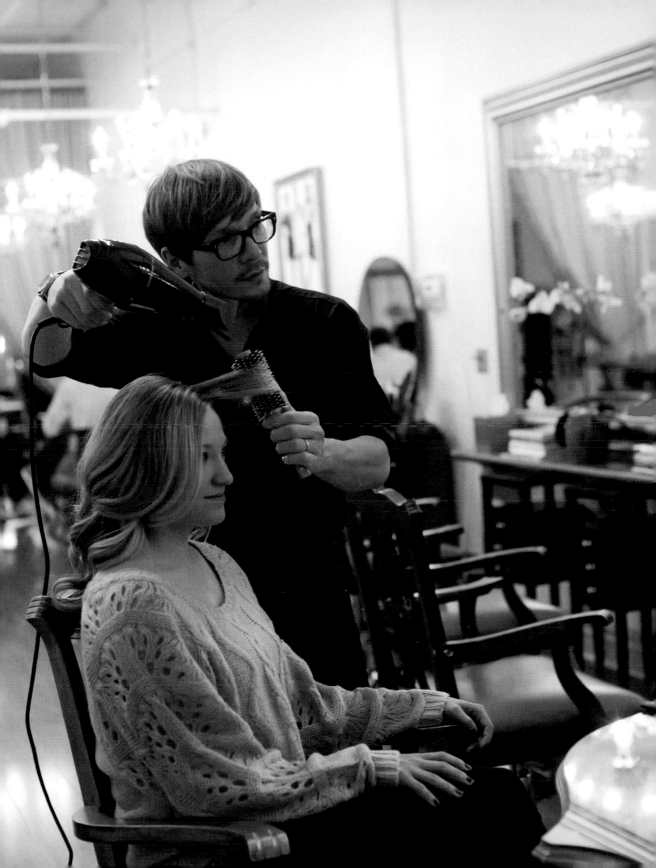

The Beauty of Cool Air

Warm air does an astonishing job of altering the texture and shape of hair—from thick, curly, and coarse to sleek and smooth; or from fine, flat, and straight to full and voluminous. Whether you are using a flat brush to smooth your hair or a round brush to add volume, heat creates the shape, but *cooling* the hair will lock it into place.

Have you ever noticed that when you've finished blow-drying your hair smooth, it swells up moments afterward—or watched the volume you've just created deflate right before your eyes?

- Try cool air to lock your style in place. Once you've achieved the desired texture for each section of your hair and while your hair is still warm and on your brush, either hold it in place while it cools or blast it with a shot of cold air (provided your dryer has a cool air button).

- Warm air opens the cuticle, helping you to change the shape of your hair; cool air closes the cuticle, locking in the newly created shape.

Hair-Care Rx

Healthy, shiny hair is the basis for any great style. When you don't take good care of your hair, it lets you know. I'm going to address hair repair a bit more before we get to all the fun styling tips because it's so important. You can have a great haircut or hairstyle, but if your hair is dry and damaged, so is your style! Let's get pretty, ladies.

It's Crunch Time

When a client or makeover candidate comes to me with hair so parched it looks crunchy to the touch, or like a steel wool pad after scouring a sinkful of pans, I ask a lot of questions to find out exactly what she's done to stress out her tresses. The two most common causes of hair damage are overwashing and overstyling. That means too much hair drying, flat ironing, and curling—basically too much fighting with the kind of hair you have.

If you learn to work with your hair's natural texture, it won't be such a struggle to keep it healthy and looking good. But if you fight to completely change the texture of your hair every time you style it, or if you are addicted to chemical processing to change it, your hair will simply rebel and keep acting up.

It's fine to use relaxers, perms, and some straightening products to create a more manageable texture. To me that's like coloring your hair. Thankfully, there are modern ways to "relax" your hair that won't destroy it, like the relaxers of yesteryear.

I've noticed that some of my friends and clients, who had previously relaxed their hair, are now growing it out, wearing it more "natural," and opting for more conditioning instead, because it offers more options, versatility, and ease of styling.

Timing Your Trims

If you're trying to grow your hair out and are afraid of trims, then keep it healthy and you will need fewer trims. Hair that breaks and splits at the ends needs constant trimming to keep up with the damage you're doing. Sorry if you don't like what I am about to say, but split ends are your fault. Keep the ends healthy and hydrated and you will require fewer trims.

I have seen many women whose hair is so damaged and dry that it literally "cuts" itself. I have also seen many chemical cuts, as we call them in the hair biz—hair that has broken off due to too much chemical processing.

If your hair is in poor condition, I recommend cutting off the damaged hair and asking your hairdresser to give you a shorter style than the one

If your hair is severely damaged or if you have coarse, curly, kinky hair that is frizzy by nature, you have to step things up a notch. Deep condition your hair on a regular basis and try to find a conditioner geared to your specific texture. You can also try using my olive oil treatments once a week (see page 72), skip blow-drying and overwashing, and get regular trims. If you have the time, there are alternatives to blow-drying your hair. For example, wet setting, wrapping damp hair, and then sitting under the dryer is a more gentle way to change the texture of your hair.

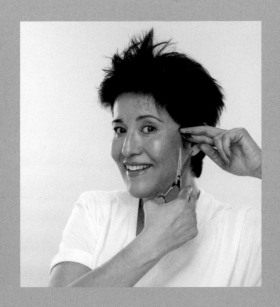

you currently have. Shorter, healthier, shiny hair is far more attractive than long, dry, dull hair that tapers off, leaving a few see-through strands at the bottom. Cutting your hair to a healthier length will also give you a chance to try a new look and an opportunity to break old, damaging habits.

Once you're practicing a healthy hair routine, I recommend cutting your hair three to four times a year, if it's long, and six to eight times a year, if it is shorter.

Chemical Processes

Less is more when it comes to chemical processes. Your hair can become a big, crazy mess if you're overlapping different chemical processes, which can destroy your hair and wreak havoc on your scalp.

Some stylists treat every chemical process like it's a virgin application by doing hair from roots to end, every single time. On the flip side, clients often think they need to have all their hair freshened up from the roots to the ends every time they go to the salon. The same goes for those of you who color, perm, or straighten your hair at home. You don't need to do your entire head every time. If the ends of your hair look drab and dull, toning your hair color on the ends with a semipermanent or deposit-only color is a better option.

Cosmetic Chemist Alec Batis on Taking Care of Chemically Treated Hair

The most important thing to do for relaxed, permed, colored, and other types of chemically treated hair is to strengthen it with products that contain plant proteins, such as soy and amino acids. But don't overtreat your hair with protein-based products. The proteins in these products—especially wheat proteins—can leave too much of a buildup on your hair, leaving it stiff, crunchy, and brittle, just as overconditioning can leave you with greasy, limp hair.

How often should you use protein-based products? It all depends on your hair. Everyone's hair is different, and as Ken says, you have to get to know your hair's type and texture, its needs, and what works for you. You will know when it's time to stop.

I always tell clients to ease up on the damaging effects of any kind of chemical processing by refreshing the roots only and not overlapping the product on areas of their hair that have been previously done. This will give your hair a break. Only address the areas that need touching up. If a straightening treatment, perm, color, or highlights are growing out, give hair that was previously done a break, since it's already been processed. Overlapping some processes or products can cause serious breakage. Make sure to discuss whether or not certain processes can be done on the same day with your stylist, in order to avoid severely damaging your hair and irritating your scalp.

Permanent color lifts the pigments out of your hair before depositing and creating a new color. Bleach and highlights also lift the pigment out of your hair. Semipermanent color and deposit-only toners add color

Taking care of chemically treated hair is complex. I recommend a three-step approach:

1. Mild cleansing (with a nonsulfate shampoo).

2. Protecting the color from water with conditioners containing at least two or three ingredients that include "quat" somewhere in the word—such as polyquaternium-87. These ingredients smooth the surface of the hair, repel water, help retain color, and make hair easier to comb, while preserving volume. You don't want to count on silicones alone to smooth your hair.

3. Protecting your color from the sun. UVA and UVB radiation damage hair and hair color, resulting in faded color and off-tone color changes. Use a leave-in conditioner that has UV protection.

to your hair without lifting it. When you get your hair highlighted, for example, stylists often apply a toner to soften and blend highlights, even a tone, or enhance a color. Toner also helps you to achieve the most flattering color for your complexion (although it is not always necessary).

Toner fades after five or more washings. When you get your roots touched up with color, your stylist may apply a toner to freshen the color.

For All You Styling Tool Addicts Out There

Unless I'm getting a client ready for the red carpet or a photo shoot, I focus on everyday glamour and beauty. So should you. I want you to find a styling regimen that makes your hair look gorgeous every day, without all the extra frying, baking, and broiling you're doing to your already overworked tresses.

By all means, if you have a special event to attend—a birthday party, an anniversary dinner, a reunion, a hot date—get out those hot rollers or that flat iron you love so much. These are the few instances when I give you carte blanche to do whatever the heck you want to do with your hair so that you'll feel like a million bucks on that special day. Healthy hair will make your style look even better for these special occasions.

But if you're overusing styling tools every day, you're not working with your hair texture—you're fighting it—which will only lead to more damage. You need to find a happy medium: a look you like and can live with every day that doesn't require overheating your hair.

Après-Workout Hair-Care Tips

Many women ask me what to do with their hair after working out, especially if they exercise every day or most days.

Most women can't wait to get in the shower and wash their hair when it feels dirty and sweaty. Once again, you don't want to overwash your hair, which will dry it out. After a particularly grueling workout, simply rinse sweaty hair with warm water. Massage your scalp with your fingers to get rid of excess oil or shampoo the roots only. Condition your hair to leave it looking and feeling fresh without dehydrating it.

If you're not dripping in sweat or don't have time for a shower, try a dry shampoo or shake a little baby powder onto your roots to soak up excess oils and sweat, which will revive freshly worked-out hair.

You can also just put your hair in a high ponytail or a low chignon for a great postworkout look.

Baby, It's Cold Outside!

Caring for your hair in the cold winter months is critical. In the fall and winter, especially in the more frigid parts of the country, the two biggest culprits women face are static, which is the result of dehydrated hair, and hair that gets oily from "hat head."

Just like your skin, your hair gets dry, flaky, and dull during the cold weather months, when you're probably using your blow-dryer even more, so that you don't have to go outside in freezing weather with wet or damp hair and catch a cold. In addition, we're essentially using a blow-dryer to keep our houses and offices warm. Heat from furnaces and other heating units dehydrates hair and skin and causes static.

Extra conditioning will keep your hair healthy when the thermometer plummets. Condition your hair every time you wash it. Deep condition your hair every week or every two weeks, either in the shower or by applying a deep conditioning mask for a half hour or so and then showering. If you are deep conditioning in the shower, leave the conditioner on for as long as you can to maximize its moisturizing benefits.

Wearing a hat or covering your head to keep warm in the cold can leave your head a little sweaty, even though your hair is dryer than usual. If you find that your scalp is oilier than normal, I recommend washing your hair every other day, if you can stand it. If you must wash your hair, remember to clean only the roots and apply conditioner just from the midshaft of your hair to your ends. This will help minimize a sweaty and oily scalp.

Another way to keep your hair hydrated in the fall and winter is to sleep with a humidifier. The lack of moisture in the air literally creates a desert-like environment in your house. This means you are living in a constant state of dehydration that severely affects your hair, skin, and nails. A humidifier will put much-needed moisture back into the air—and you just might wake up looking younger.

Hair Care in the Sizzling Summertime

Oddly enough, the remedies for both cold and extremely hot and humid climates are almost exactly the same: hydration and conditioning.

Typically, you spend more time outdoors in the warm summer months, which means that your hair is more exposed to the damaging rays of the sun, chlorine in pools, and salt in ocean water—all of which dehydrate hair. You also tend to sweat more. These factors, plus extra dirt and environmental debris, warrant extra shampooing, which can destroy hair. On top of that, of course, are the hazards of frying and burning hair with flat irons, curling irons, and blow-dryers to combat summertime frizz.

In addition to conditioning your hair every time you shampoo and giving your hair regular deep conditioning, I always tell my clients to wet their hair and apply conditioner before jumping in the pool. Once your hair's in the water, the cuticles open up and absorb chlorine, which can leave your hair dry and ratty-looking. If you wet your hair first and apply conditioner, your cuticles soak up the conditioner instead of the chlorine. When you're done swimming, always rinse your hair with clean water, if you can. Tuck a bottle of your favorite conditioner in your beach bag and apply it after you rinse your hair. Look for some of the great products that protect your hair against ultraviolet rays and chlorine.

As I've said earlier, try not to overshampoo your hair in the hot summer months. Do not wash it every day. Rinse with warm water and condition from the midshaft to the ends.

Take Advantage of the Heat

Summertime heat opens the cuticle of your hair. Why not exploit this natural warmth to help condition and protect it? Just coat your damp hair with an even distribution of your favorite conditioner or treatment, then pull it back into a ponytail, wrap it into a chignon, or braid it. Getting your hair off your neck will feel cool and comfortable, and your new style will also look chic!

And since it's summer, air-dry your hair as much as you can. Get in your car, roll down all the windows or put the top down, and let nature do the drying for you. It will save your hair. I promise.

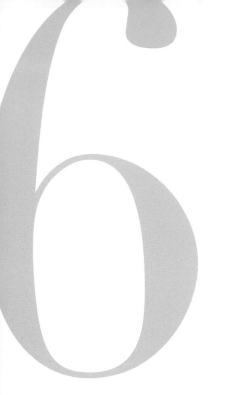

Your Best Accessory

Just as the confidence you exude lets the world know how beautiful and significant you are, so does the way you feel about your hair.

For centuries, hair has been synonymous with beauty and femininity. Your hair is your crowning glory. Whatever kind of hair you have, wear it like a crown. Treat it well and find the best cut and style for your hair type and texture, personality, and lifestyle. When you feel great about your hair, everything else about your look seems to work. Everyone knows how fantastic you feel when you're having "a good hair day."

It's a psychological thing. You could be wearing jeans, a T-shirt, and flip-flops, but if your hair looks great and you feel good about it, you're going to feel beautiful. That's because hair is different from everything else when it comes to your looks. Makeup can be applied. You can change your clothes and your jewelry, depending on where you're going that day or to suit your mood. Unless you've lost your hair to illness (like my dear friend, Sarah Lucero, who lost hers to chemotherapy treatments but still looks gorgeous!), it's the one physical attribute you have that can instantly make you feel great inside and out. That's why your hair is your best accessory!

Once again, this all goes back to accepting yourself, understanding who you are, keeping current with yourself, and making the most of what you've got to feel your best. When you feel good about who you are as a person and see the positive results that come from taking care of yourself, you automatically feel better. Celebrate yourself!

Sarah's Story

"In November 2010, I noticed a lump in my right breast," says my amazing and beautiful friend, Sarah Lucero. *"It was painful and getting bigger every day. I figured it was a cyst that needed draining or something like that.*

"I had a mammogram to see what I was dealing with and will never forget what happened that day. I arrived for an early appointment and was told I needed an ultrasound. As I lay on the ultrasound table, I knew in my gut that something was not right. It took a really long time to complete the ultrasound. Then a doctor walked into the room. She said the lump was not a cyst and she thought it could be breast cancer. A biopsy was done immediately and I went home. The doctor called me the next day to tell me I had breast cancer.

"At that moment, I felt so many emotions and didn't even know how to react or what to do. I don't think anything can prepare you for news like this. I somehow remained very calm and very focused during the next few weeks, planning for my treatments and meeting with several doctors.

I did not tell very many people about my cancer, since I knew I needed to focus all of my energy—mental and physical—on getting better.

"I felt like it was hardest to tell the people closest to me that I had cancer. I didn't want them to worry about me or look at me differently. I'm so grateful and thankful for all my friends and family who helped me get through the toughest days. I'm most thankful and grateful that I was able to keep a positive attitude during this time of my life. What I thought would be the worst thing for me actually turned out to be one of the best things for me.

"I work in the beauty industry, as the global creative director for Stila Cosmetics. I had booked several TV segments for the red carpet season and was going to be on the air. I knew I would lose my hair and was told to get a wig before it fell out. In fact, the chemotherapy made all of my hair fall out after the very first treatment.

"Of course I felt sad about losing my beautiful hair. I tried to focus on keeping a positive and brave attitude about it. I learned very quickly to let go and accept the things that I had no control over. That's how I dealt with everything during my treatment. I only dealt with what was right in front of me at that moment and did not look beyond or think of what-ifs.

"I experienced many amazing blessings while I was sick. One of the greatest blessings was becoming close friends with Ken Paves. I got to know Ken through our client and good friend, Victoria Beckham. After Victoria found out I had cancer, she asked Ken to make me a wig since she knew how much it would mean to me to look like myself again and to feel beautiful inside and out. That was so kind of Victoria and Ken. I will be forever grateful to them both for caring about me so much and wanting to help me.

"Ken—and Alexis from his salon— worked on making the most gorgeous wig that looked exactly like my old hair . . . except way better! The first time I put it on at Ken's salon was so exciting. When I looked into the mirror I looked like myself again for the first time in so long. I will never forget that moment. Ken helped me feel beautiful and confident again.

"I have had many laughs and many tears with Ken. He is one of the most inspirational, selfless, generous, kind, positive, loving, and caring people I've ever met. He makes me laugh so much. I never felt sick when I was around him. Ken has a special gift that allows him to brighten your day with his smile. He believed in me and gave me hope, happiness, and gorgeous hair!"

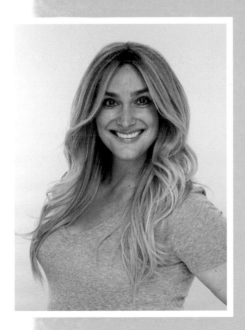 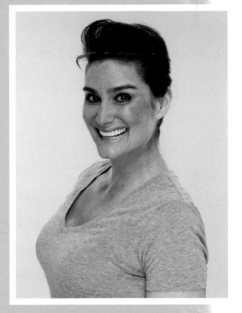

Just as beautiful! **LEFT**: Sarah, wearing the long wig I created for her.
RIGHT: Sarah's sexy short hair, styled into a cool pompadour.

Choosing the Right Style for Your Best Features

Hair is like a picture frame around your face. It can accentuate the areas you like best and crop out those that you don't. A lot of women say they think their eyes or lips are their best feature. When you're thinking about changing your hairstyle, focus on the features you like best and showcase them with face-framing haircuts, color, and texture. Ask your stylist to tailor a style that will highlight the features that make you feel the most beautiful.

If You Love Your Eyes

There are so many ways to play up your eyes with gorgeous bangs—long or short—or with face-framing layers, which will bring all the focus to your eyes.

You can also accentuate your eyes with color. Darkening your hair or adding depth to your hair with a deeper shade of color brings focus to your eyes by creating a frame around your face. Lightness lifts attention up and away from the face. Depth draws everything closer in. If you're painting a room, for example, dark-colored molding gives the illusion of bringing the ceiling down and into the room, giving it a cozy feel. On the other hand, light-colored molding makes a room seem bigger and more expansive. It moves everything up and away from the room.

To bring attention to your eyes, bring the frame of your hair in closer to your face. One of the things I do to accentuate a woman's eyes is to apply the deepest shade I'm using to color her hairline. I use a thin line of color—a quarter inch or so from the hairline back, across the entire hairline—to give the illusion of bringing the hair in tighter toward the face.

If you're blonde and have a deeper blonde base color and lighter blonde highlights, for example, make sure that a quarter inch of your entire hairline has the deeper blonde on it to highlight your eyes. Don't apply highlights to the perimeter, which will break the illusion of the frame around the face.

If You Love Your Lips

Bring all the interest to your lips with flattering, face-framing layers. A beautiful jawline or chin-length cut will make it all about your mouth. A bob or face-framing layers that fall downward toward the chin will also accentuate your sexy pout.

If You Love Your Cheekbones

To accentuate your cheekbones, you want to lift your hair up and away from your face. One great way to do this is with layers that pull back and open up your face to let the world see those gorgeous cheekbones you so love. Hair that's curled away from the face opens it up and lifts up the jawline. Hair that's blown back and away from the face does the same thing.

You can also style your hair to accentuate your cheekbones. Layers are so great because they enable you to direct your hair any way you want it to go, whether the layers are flowing back away from your face or styled forward toward your face. Curling layers of hair back and away from the face, as I have done for Eva Longoria and Jessica Simpson, will give you an effortless, contemporary look. (I'll show you a variety of curling techniques from retro to Boho chic on page 184.) Make sure to keep the styling modern, though. If you curl everything toward your face, you could go eighties real quick!

If You Love Your Neck or Jawline

A taut, firm jawline gives the illusion of strength and youth. Short hair is amazing for women who have a strong jawline or a swanlike neck. A cropped cut or a cut that tapers in toward the neck will also show off these areas beautifully. So will a bob.

Longhaired women who love their neck and jawline can show off these areas by wearing their hair back, like Jennifer Lopez often does.

Victoria Beckham has a feminine neck and a great jawline and looks fantastic with a variety of short hairstyles. Now that she has grown her hair long, Victoria often wears it pulled back, which also accentuates these areas beautifully.

If You Love Your Hairline

Opt for a beautiful cut that you can tuck behind your ears to show off your beautiful hairline, whether it's high or low, and avoid bangs, which will hide your hairline.

Accepting Yourself...in the Now

Maybe you read this last section, hightailed it to your salon, and asked for a cut to show off your best feature or features. Fantastic! I have to say, though, that getting women—and men—to tell me what their favorite features are isn't always so easy.

What I have found over the years with many makeover candidates, especially those who have lost a lot of weight, like the *Biggest*

Loser contestants, is that even after significant weight loss, they often still see themselves as the heavy person they once were, making it difficult for them to recognize their favorite features. They become so used to not liking what they see that it is hard for them to get beyond that memory and embrace how amazing they look today. This is the case with many people—whether they see themselves in a positive or negative way, it is often still an image from the past.

I always encourage people to focus on the attributes that they like about themselves, although they often still see only what they don't like. When you focus on the negative—everything you don't like about yourself year after year—sometimes that's all you can see when you look in the mirror.

Part of my job is to help people recognize and accept themselves in the now, to believe in the positive and to celebrate who they are in this moment! In some cases, that meant dramatically changing the looks of *The Biggest Loser* contestants so when they looked in the mirror afterward, they no longer saw their former selves but rather the slimmed-down, healthier, beautiful person they had worked so hard to become.

You, dear reader, have to get to this point as well. There has to be something that you love about your features when you look in the mirror. It goes back to accepting yourself, embracing who you are in this moment, and believing that you deserve to feel beautiful.

Even so, I can't tell you how many times I've asked women in my chair to tell me what they like best about themselves so I can give them the best cut possible, and the first thing I hear is what they don't like. One of my clients actually told me that she hated her "whole face!" My reaction was to joke with her: "Uhhhhh…that's going to make things tough for me because I can't just pull a ponytail in front of your face and leave it there forever." She laughed and we ended up finding the perfect cut for her that was easy to maintain and brought out the best in her. (She finally admitted that she loves her smile.) Sometimes being able to laugh "with" yourself brings out the truth.

Stop Living in the Past

I also find that when I ask the women who sit in my chair to look in the mirror and tell me what they love about what they see, many of them tell me, "There's so much I *used* to love." That harsh self-criticism makes it harder for women to accept who they are right now.

One woman told me she hated the way her face looked because "everything was older than it was before." Surely there was something there she liked, I said. She finally admitted that she loved her eyes, but she made sure to let me know that she didn't love her eyelids or the skin around her eyes. Basically, she loved her eyeballs. But that's OK. It was a start.

I understood where my client was coming from. She felt that she had matured a lot and that her skin looked a lot different than it used to look when she was in her twenties, thirties, and even forties. The interesting thing is that this woman had taken to wearing hats for several years. I don't know if she intentionally wore them to camouflage her eyes, but anytime you wear a hat it puts a shadow over the face that can soften the appearance of wrinkles around the eyes.

I used the same theory when I cut her hair. For this particular woman, I ended up cutting a long fringe that came just below her eyebrows, accentuating her gorgeous brown eyes while camouflaging the eyelids she disliked so much. I colored her hair a deep, rich red-brown. The color alone was a statement and, oddly enough, just like a great hat it distracted the eye from the features she didn't like underneath it. When we were finished, she told me she felt more beautiful than she had in a long time.

Beauty Is Always Evolving

All too often, women sporting the same hairdo they had in high school look in the mirror and are somehow surprised by a face that is clearly not in high school anymore looking back at them! If this is you, you are setting yourself up for disappointment. If you're expecting a teenage face to look back at you, you're not being fair to yourself.

> You don't ever want to look like a vintage version of yourself. A vintage handbag is great…a vintage you, not so much!

If you are unhappy with what you see in the mirror because it reminds you of the past, then it's important at some point in your life to change things and get as far away from where you were before so that you can see how beautiful you are now.

My Own Journey with Evolving Looks

I came to an important realization about my own looks a few years ago when I started looking at myself, particularly in photos, and realized that I didn't feel like "that" person anymore. I had evolved on the inside and wanted to recognize those changes on the outside. Change doesn't necessarily mean that something is better, but growth is certainly good for the soul.

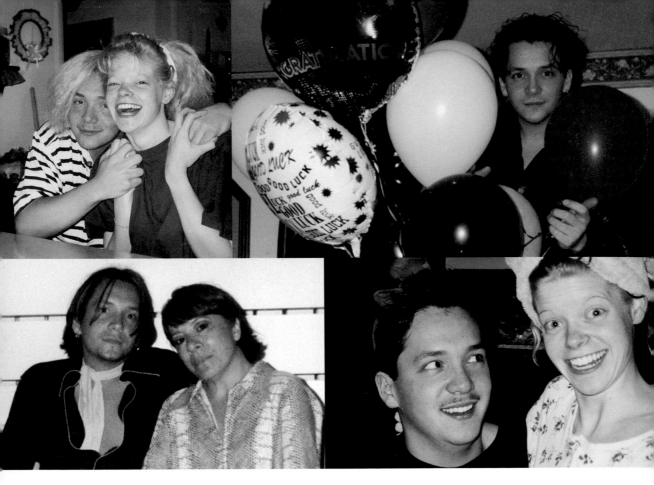

Clockwise from top left: me, dreaming of one day having Audrey's blonde hair;
I actually graduated from beauty school with a black permed bob; my natural hair and
"college 15" (pounds); Mom and me, living it up in Miami. I love a tan!

I was very blond at the time, as I had been for years. My natural hair color is dark brown. When I looked in the mirror, though, my blond hair reminded me of who I used to be. I felt like I was looking at the "old" me. I wanted to see the present me. I didn't see the man I'd become, from all the amazing experiences I'd had, nurturing my mind and soul. I had neglected to bring my reflection up to date.

I changed my hair back to its natural brown and loved it. I feel good about where I've come from and where I've arrived. I recognize the man in the mirror and I like who I see—me.

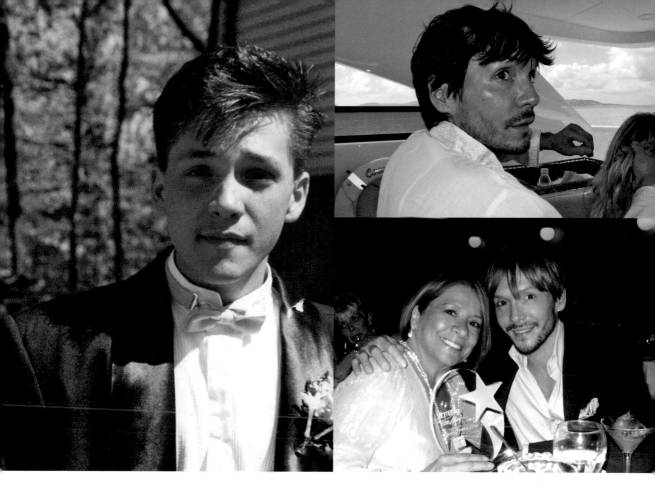

Clockwise from left: my junior prom, channeling the movie *Sixteen Candles*; my natural hair in St. Bart's; Mother and son, same hair color. Mom won a philanthropy award that night.

When you truly accept yourself, by your own standards, everyone else seems to follow. Self-acceptance becomes attractive to other people. If everybody could just look in the mirror and smile and see a loving, accepting friend smiling back, things would be easier for everyone. That's the best way to start your day—happy to see a familiar friend.

Does this mean that I'm happy with every single thing about myself? No. But I've accepted who I am and I'm loving getting to know myself day by day. If that means I may be blond again tomorrow, then so be it. Living is all about being present with yourself, in *this* amazing moment. It's okay to revisit that past, but it's not okay to be stuck there.

It's Not the Eighties Anymore

My good friend Elan Bongiorno is a talented celebrity makeup artist for stars like Eva Longoria and Jane Fonda. She is the founder of Enjoué Beauté cosmetics. She's in her forties now and always tells me and Eva, "You should have seen my ass in the eighties! My ass was up here!"

Whenever she brings this up, I joke, "Well, guess what? It's not the eighties anymore and I hate to tell you but your ass isn't up to there anymore!" Elan laughs—and is able to laugh at herself because she has a great connection to reality. Yes, she knows her body isn't the same as it was many years ago. She knows she has changed physically—and she's all right with that. Elan is still a beautiful woman, inside and out. These days she focuses on what makes her feel good on the inside. She volunteers her time to the Beauty Bus Foundation and Haven Hills Domestic Violence Shelter, helping to empower other women and make them feel confident and beautiful. In return, this makes Elan feel good about herself. In this attitude she is vastly differ- ent from a woman who is down on herself now because she doesn't look like she used to look. No one does. Elan is a perfect example of living and loving yourself in this moment.

When you base your self-esteem on your beauty, you only set yourself up for disappointment.

The flip side of this is that many women look better now than they did when they were younger. Sure, things might've been perkier and tighter then and their skin might have had a more youthful glow, but, as women grow older, they radiate a life's worth of confidence that allows their inner beauty to shine.

Now You See It, Now You Don't

You've earned every wrinkle and laugh line on your face. Right? But just in case you don't absolutely love them all, here are some tips and tricks to camouflage areas you may not want to show the world, including wrinkles on your forehead, acne, and a maturing neck. Yes, I have said throughout this book to accept yourself for who you are right now, but if you can downplay features you aren't so thrilled about, thus helping you accept and feel better about who you are and what you look like, then why not?

As you have seen, hair is like a frame that can be used to accentuate the features you love and crop out those that you don't. And with the right products and care, hair can be made to look luxurious, healthy, and vibrant, bringing the focus of the eye to your locks and not to a particular feature you don't like.

When camouflaging with hair, focus on the facial features you love, and use hair to distract from those you don't love. Here are a few tips that work beautifully:

- Bangs, fringe, and face-framing layers can cover up acne, wrinkles on the forehead, scars, crow's-feet, and other fine lines.

- If your eyes are a concern, you can opt for a stronger perimeter haircut—an asymmetrical or choppy bob, which draws attention away from the eyes and to a different focal point on your face or neck.

- Parting the hair to one side can camouflage and hide a

droopy eye with a long bang or fringe.

♦ Layers can do wonders for covering up features you don't want to emphasize. Some women blow their hair slightly in toward the face. Directing the hair closer in to the face can bring attention to the eyes or lips, depending on how you style it, while camouflaging a double chin or lines around the eyes.

♦ Another place for some nice camouflaging layers is the area between the cheek and ear, which can look crepe-like as women get older.

♦ If a woman is self-conscious about her neck, she can wear bangs to bring attention to the eyes to distract from the neck. If her hair is shoulder-length or longer, cutting the hair in layers will also camouflage the neck area.

Shake It Up!

When I'm cutting or styling a woman's hair, I like to keep things versatile. You're so limited when you have only one option with your hair. What many people notice about my work with my celebrity clients is that I am always able to create different looks based on a client's particular style. You should be able to do this too.

You probably know all too well how hair can differ from day to day. Sometimes it does what it wants. You will struggle with it a lot less if you can do different things with it.

I tailor a cut individually for each client, ensuring that it is versatile for her. A cut is versatile when it allows you to wear your hair parted to one side one day and parted to the other side the next. It's versatile when you can wear it with a nondescript parting, blown out smooth, wavy, or curly. A versatile cut will be forgiving if you can't devote much time to styling your hair. We all know a cut never looks exactly the same as when you leave the salon, but it should still look beautiful!

I do all different kinds of haircutting and once studied a philosophy of haircutting that was all about severe, straight lines and definitive partings. This was nice in theory but not so great in reality. If the wind blew and a woman's hair accidentally parted to the other side, she ended up with a long piece hanging over the other side of her head. Not so pretty.

When choosing a cut, you want to look for something you can easily wear up or down or straight or curly, depending on your mood and how much time you have to style it. Whatever cut you choose, it should fit your hair texture and type as well as your lifestyle. If it's a versatile cut, you should be able to blow it out or smooth it out for a sleek look and wear it just as well with a curl or wave. And if the wind blows your hair, it will still look great.

What *real women* have to say about . . .

Their Hair

"Since my hair is a little naturally curly, I like to straighten it," says Sarah M. *"It's simple and matches my facial features. I go between curly and straight. I like to keep it fresh and natural as much as possible. Sometimes I'll do a pony. My favorite quick look is putting it in a ballerina bun on top of my head. I like to use a spin pin. You spin it and it gives you a two-second updo."*

"I love my hair short," says Chloe. *"I've worn it short for about thirty-five years. I've tried to grow it out but I felt older and matronly and*

unfashionable. As soon as I cut my hair short, I come to life again. It exposes my face, my neck, and my shoulders. I feel lighter. I'll wear it up or slicked down. I put tons of product in it so it looks distressed—if your hair is too soft when it's short, it just limps down. I don't condition because I have short hair and it won't get damaged because I'm always cutting it."

"When I was in my mid-forties, Ken went to beauty school and everything changed," says Helen. *"I became his guinea pig, and I loved it. He automatically took me from a spiral perm to a classic A-line bob, which we permed straight to start fresh. This is when all my hair-coloring changes started as well. Up until then I had always colored my hair medium brown out of a box. I was a do-it-yourself girl. Ken then gave me a caramel-colored bob, a pixie cut, and a chestnut-brown shag with highlighted edges. I also had a dark honey-blonde bob variation. I remember he gave me three cuts in one night until my husband said, 'OK. Stop. Your mother looks great.' In my fifties, I had everything. I had a short, layered, caramel flip; I had an all-one-length, shoulder-skimming chocolate-brown style; I've had bangs and no bangs; and I had a short blonde pixie when I met Celine Dion for my fifty-eighth birthday.*

"Ken opened our Michigan salon when I was fifty-seven, so since then I have tried out even more cuts, colors, and even extensions. I started with Ken's HairDo extensions and, later, fused-in extensions. Now that I am in my sixties, I have a short bob again. I guess what is old is new again. Last week my bob was brown and A-line and Ken just made it shorter. It's cropped in the back and caramel-colored with blonde tips. What's next?"

Big Bang Theory

Whether you're trying to accentuate a feature or downplay it, bangs are one of the best ways to do this. Bangs work for almost everyone. They give even the simplest hairstyle some personality. They can create softness around the face and give you many different opportunities for hairstyling.

Most women say they love a style with bangs because it makes them look younger. Bangs can instantly take years off a woman's face. Bangs are also the ultimate for anybody who is in a transitional phase with a cut. Bangs are the most forgiving and quickest way to create a new look.

Bangs are always a go-to look because they are so versatile, which is how I can customize a look for a particular woman. You can choose a sweeping bang or bangs that go straight across the forehead. And bangs can be parted on either side of the face—they don't always have to be dead center. In fact, they can be askew, which gives a casual, flirtatious look.

I love a deep, side-parted bang for a dramatic, severe look. This is where you part the hair furthest

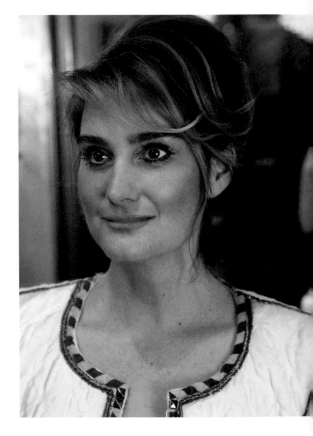

Sarah L. wearing her Bardot-inspired bangs, side swept.

from either side. I've done this with Victoria Beckham quite a few times. The end result is stunning.

One of the looks my clients request most is the "Bardot bang," which is one of my favorite cuts. Inspired by the 1960s sex symbol Brigitte Bardot (who had oodles of confidence!), this kind of bang is short in the center and longer on the sides.

The Bardot bang is one of the most versatile kinds of bangs because you can wear it to the side, with a sexy fringe covering one side of the face. You can also part the hair in the middle, with hair falling to both sides of the face for an übersexy look every single day.

You often see women with a long piece of hair swept over to one side of the face. That's still considered a bang. It's a side-swept bang. It just lies a little differently. You still cut it using the bang technique, but you cut it longer so a woman can wear it casually or more "done."

Choosing the Right Bang

When selecting a bang, you and your stylist have to take a few things into consideration:

- what look you are hoping for

- how the hair grows in on your hairline, above your forehead

- what you want to accentuate or camouflage

- how you like to style your hair

- what hair texture and type you have

- how much time you want to commit to the upkeep and styling of bangs

It's all about tailoring the bang to your specific needs. Bangs that go straight across the forehead might not work for everyone. The beauty of bangs is that you can cut so many variations of them to suit your particular look, hair texture, and type. That's when it gets fun and creative.

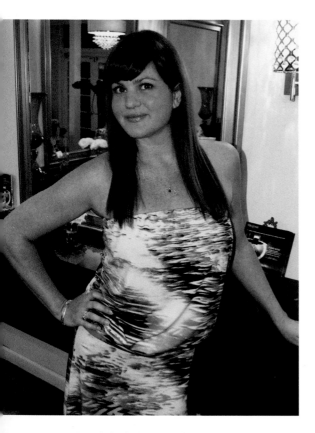

People had always told Tip she shouldn't wear bangs because of her "face shape." Not so. I think she looks great!

Bangs for Everyone!

It used to be said that a person with a full face could not wear bangs. Not the case. If you have a full face, choose a bang that showcases the highest point of your forehead. When you can see the highest point of a woman's forehead and the lowest point of the chin, it gives a visual illusion that elongates and narrows the face. Bardot-style bangs parted down the center and side-swept bangs are great options to achieve this look.

This is a perfect example of why I don't subscribe to those so-called tenets about face shape, which I will explore in depth later on (see page 126). You can have any bang or cut you want, as long as it's tailored to your particular needs.

Many stylists say a woman can't have bangs because she has a "round" or "square" face. Boring! Don't want to hear it! Sounds like an excuse to me. If you have a full face, you have more facial real estate, which is even more reason to contour it with a great set of customized bangs. Your stylist just has to work harder and think out of the box.

The Curly-Haired Conundrum

Another myth is that women with curly hair can't have bangs. Not so. A layered haircut with curly bangs is a beautiful option. Toni Braxton shows off one of the most classic examples of curly hair with curly bangs in her video for her hit song, "Unbreak My Heart." You can wear the bangs curly or smooth them out, depending on the look you're seeking.

Curly, layered hair with bangs can sometimes evoke a retro, seventies shag feeling. Beyoncé has done it. Minnie Driver has done it. I styled her hair for years and we did curly bangs that looked fantastic.

How to Cut Your Own Bangs

Sometimes you might not have the time or cash to pop into the salon for a bang trim. Or you may be tired of hair that lies flat and lifeless along the sides of your face and you want a change—fast. In this section, I will teach you how to cut your own bangs easily and accurately.

When I mention to some women that yes, they can easily cut their own bangs, they act as though I have asked them to perform surgery on themselves. "No way, Ken! If I cut my own hair, it would be a disaster." Not really. You will be surprised by how easy it is to cut bangs if you've never done it before. They're a lot more forgiving than you think.

To be honest, bangs you cut yourself might not be as technically perfect as when you have them done professionally at the salon, but they can still look great. Plus, I feel imperfections evoke a casual elegance and lessen the stress to be "perfect." Some of my least "perfect" haircuts look the best.

Start With the Right Tools

You'll need good lighting, a mirror, a comb, a couple of hair clips or a ponytail holder, and scissors. If you don't have haircutting scissors, choose a pair that is small and manageable.

Preparing to Cut a Bang

The number-one mistake most women make when doing their own bangs is cutting deep into hair that isn't meant to come forward into a bang. This will leave you with short hair where you don't want it. Here's how to avoid this mistake:

- Before you cut a single strand, you need to determine where the hair is that will fall forward into the bang and how far back you want to cut it.

- No matter where you normally part your hair, part it down the middle to get the hair to fall evenly on both sides.

Cut bangs on dry hair only

When cutting bangs yourself, I recommend doing it on dry hair so that you achieve an accurate length and get a truer picture of what the bangs will look like when you're finished.

Wet hair stretches more than dry hair. This is where error comes in. If you cut your hair when it's wet, it could turn out supershort and you won't be happy with what you see in the mirror. That's when you'll be in a headband for a month until your hair starts to grow out.

Cutting curly hair yourself when it's wet is especially dangerous, because it shrinks up considerably more when it dries.

- To ensure that you don't cut into hair that won't be part of the bang, put your index finger in the middle of your forehead, bending it up and into the hairline. This will help you figure out where the top of your head begins to round down toward your forehead. The hair here tends to fall forward and easily into bangs. This area should be about an inch to an inch and a half back from your hairline.

- Once you've located this initial point in the middle of your head, use your comb to separate the hair that you want to cut into a bang, and neatly clip the rest back and out of the way. This is where a lot of women accidentally pull more of their side hair into the bangs and cut more than they intend to cut—deep back—and end up looking like they are wearing an acorn cap.

- As an extra precaution, carefully comb the soon-to-be bang area down toward the face, so you can look at the hair on each side of your head to make sure that only the hair you want to cut into a bang is hanging down and separated from the hair you don't want to snip.

- Keep in mind that hair that has been straightened will shrink considerably when it's back in its natural state. Allow plenty of room for shrinkage.

- If your hair is wavy, curly, or kinky, you may need to smooth or straighten it, with your blow-dryer and a brush, in order to get a more precise cut.

- Now that the rest of your hair is tucked away and you have the hair you want to cut hanging over your forehead, comb that bit of hair forward loosely. You want to see exactly how it falls naturally on your face. If you pull the hair down too hard, you may end up cutting more than you intended. You should begin cutting a longer length than you might want for a bang: you can always go back and trim more later.

Cutting a Straight Bang

- When cutting a straight bang, you should cut the hair straight across first, to get the basic shape and length. Look in the mirror. Comb the hair you plan to cut in front of your face. Gather all this hair into about an inch-wide section, holding the hair in place between your index and middle fingers.

- Begin cutting the hair straight across. You can start to cut below the eyebrows or even a little lower, if you wish. Gathering the hair and cutting it straight across creates a bang that looks straight, but is actually slightly longer on the outsides. This looks more modern and helps the bang to blend into the sides.

- Don't try to cut it all in one sweep. Go section by section. Release this hair and comb it back down to see how you're doing. Repeat the steps above until you achieve the desired length.

- Step back from the mirror and take another look. Decide if you want to go a little bit shorter. If so, cut straight across again, taking off just a little bit more hair. It's better to leave the bangs a little too long so that you have some left to trim rather than going too short right away.

- Once you have the initial length and shape, then you can comb your new bangs down and into place. If you're happy with the shape, you can either leave them or tailor them even more.

- I always finish bangs off by cutting them freehand. This mean you're not holding them in place. They are just falling naturally. At this point you can now trim the corners shorter if you want a more dramatic and blunt bang, or you can point cut—or chip—into your bangs for a softer look.

- Point cutting (or chipping) means you point the scissors up and slightly at an angle into the ends of your hair to lightly break up a blunt line. This gives your hair a very soft and airy look. Start on the conservative side with this technique so you do not cut too deep or change the length too much. Be very careful not to cut yourself or your eyelashes. Only do this when you can be very still, without any distractions.

Cutting a Side Bang

- Follow the directions above on how to prepare your hair for cutting bangs.

- For a side bang, decide where you want to part your hair. The width of the section of hair you want to cut should run approximately from iris to iris.

- As with the straight bang, decide where you want the bang to fall when you look at yourself in the mirror. Always go a little bit longer than that. If you want the hair to fall below the eyebrows, for instance, you would begin cutting at about the middle of your eye.

- If you want the bang to go from left to right, neatly comb the hair down in front of your face, then sweep or gather all of it to the left, a little beyond your usual part.

◆ Gather all this hair into about an inch-wide section, holding the hair in place between your index and middle fingers. Cut it straight across. This makes the hair shorter on the left and longer on the right. When you let that go, you will have the most amazing sweep across your forehead from left to right.

◆ If you want your bangs to sweep from right to left, direct all the hair completely to the right and cut the bang the same as above.

◆ If you want a side bang that's a little wispier, comb your new bang down and in place and point cut or chip into your bangs for a softer look (as described above).

Lisa, cutting a side bang

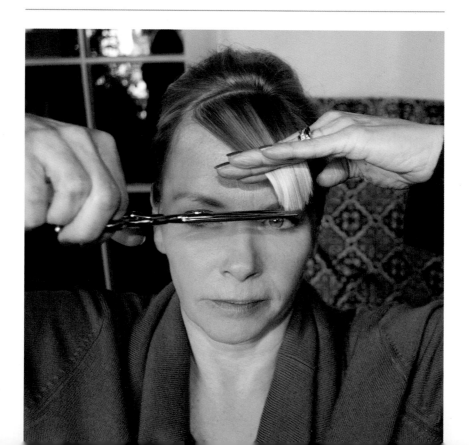

To Follow…or Not to Follow…Hair Trends

Many women go to their stylists and ask for the "hot" cut of the moment. It's great to keep on top of what looks are in. However, I like my clients to look relevant and current, rather than trendy. Trendy is getting the same haircut that seven of your friends have; trendy is when someone in the spotlight sports a great new look and everybody goes out and gets that haircut. I think it's chic to be influenced by what's happening in fashion and beauty when it comes to your look. But I don't think it's so chic to do exactly what everyone else is doing.

You don't want to wed yourself to a particular look that's in right now, especially if it's not going to work for you. You can tailor current trends to fit any style or length that suits your hair type and personality by taking elements of whatever is current about that cut and making them work for you.

Take the bob, for instance. While different versions of it are always around, the traditional bob makes a big, splashy resurgence every couple of years and has everybody running to her salon for that look. What everyone loves about a bob is that it has really clean lines and always looks fresh and new.

But before you pick up the phone to make an appointment with your stylist, think about whether this or any other cut is the right look for you. It might not be.

What you can do instead is get a blunt haircut that has the feeling of a bob with clean lines on the bottom, but isn't as short as a traditional bob. Talk to your stylist and tailor that cut to suit your own needs.

Lovely Layers

Like the bob, long layers are always in vogue, whether on short or long hair. While layers can be used to frame your face to accentuate the features you love and camouflage areas you'd like to downplay, they also add excitement to your hair. Layers give hair movement. They create texture. They add lots of personality, giving you an opportunity to find your own style.

Layers can be used to thin out and take away some of the weight of your hair, especially if it's very thick or long. They can also make hair look more voluminous and give it lots of body.

Without layers, for example, Tip's naturally wavy hair becomes very straight and almost stringy-looking. When her hair is layered, it comes alive and moves with her—and looks gorgeous.

That's why some people consider hair to be more important for a woman's look than makeup. Hair is dynamic. It moves. Makeup stays put (as you want it to), but you want your hair to react and have life. Layers help you to do that. What's key is that the layers you choose flatter you.

Sarah M.'s layers styled three different ways.

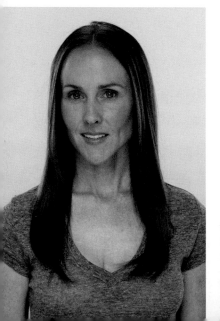
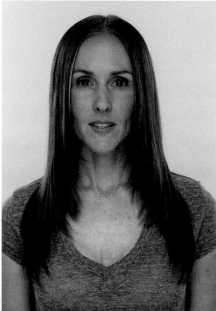
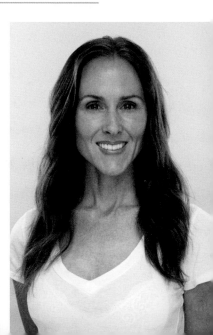

Layers come in so many variations. Take a look at these pictures of my friends Sarah M. (right) and Tip (below).

Both of them have a layered cut—but each one is different and tailored to her particular needs. Sarah has a small face, so I used layers to pull her hair up and away from her face, to open it up and make it look broader.

Tip's hair is layered around the bottom and frames her face, taking advantage of her natural waves. She lives for her waves. Her layers distract from her neck and jawline, which she considers problem areas.

Another thing I love about layers is that, depending on what's going on trend-wise, you can layer your hair ever so slightly and change it just enough to take advantage of what's happening at the moment, without becoming too trendy.

Long layering is the most forgiving and versatile way to cut hair. It works with every hair type and texture. Long-layered, sexy hair is not that far off from the layers Farrah Fawcett made so famous in the seventies. Now those layers are styled in a completely different way. For example, you could have layers that are longer and more grown out to give you a more Boho, natural vibe. Nicole Ritchie and Mary Kate and Ashley Olsen have that kind of long-layered Boho look. Sienna Miller has it as well, at times.

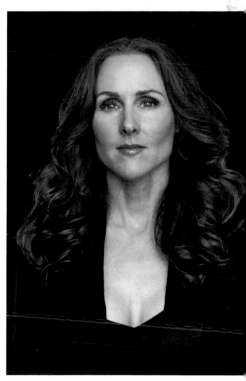

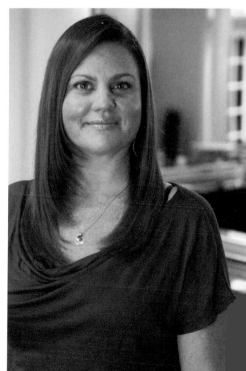

You could also opt for layers that cascade from the middle of your head—beautiful face-framing layers that get longer in the back, as so many Victoria's Secret models wear their hair.

You don't have to have long hair to have layers. Layers are what give most haircuts their individual flair. A stylist can create layers on shoulder-length hair that can look beautiful. As trends come and go, you can layer the hair a little bit shorter for a shaggier vibe.

If you have chin-length hair, all the same principles apply. Layers in short hair will give your hair movement, depending on its texture and shape.

When you discuss layers at the beauty salon, you want to make sure your stylist understands the look you hope to achieve, as well as your hair type and texture. Layers that work for curly hair don't necessarily work for straight hair. Your stylist can adjust the cut to achieve a similar look, keeping your texture in mind.

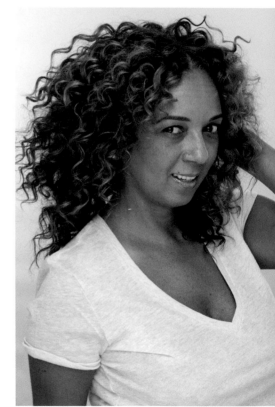

Tip has lots of beautiful waves, so we can layer her hair to give her the Farrah Fawcett look—from the crown to the ends. But if I cut that many layers on a woman with straight, fine hair, she would wind up with six straggly hairs at the bottom.

Tip, however, can never have enough layers. "Layer me, baby," she says, and when we're finished she always asks, "Can you do a little bit more?"

Charlene, with her rounded, voluminous layers

My friend Audrey has a lot of very fine, straight hair. Her hair can't be layered all over. If she layered her hair through the back, for instance, she would feel like she had even less hair. She layers it around her face only.

Charlene has great curly hair, so her layers are very rounded along the outside perimeter of her hair, so she gets tons of volume and movement without getting the dreaded "triangular" layered curly cut.

My mom has a layered A-line bob. She has graduated layers in the back of her hair and crown that create volume. Face-framing layers create a nice side fringe, which is versatile enough to be worn down the middle.

Chloe, working on Helen's bob

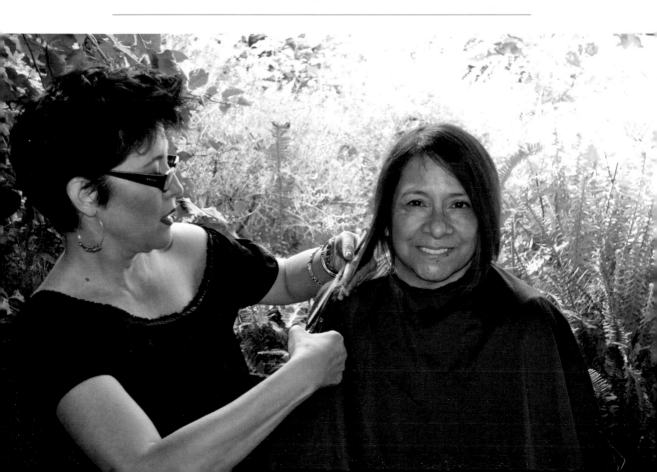

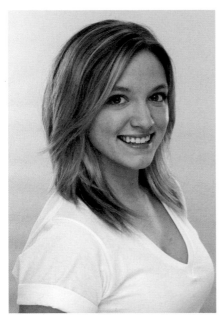

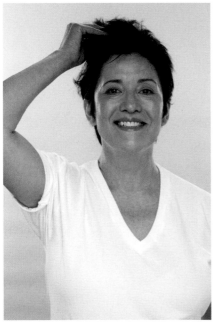

My niece Caitlin (left) has very thick hair. She may have more hair than anyone I know. She may even have more hair than Eva Longoria, who I say has enough hair for five women. Caitlin's hair is heavily layered to create movement and reduce weight. Unlike women with fine hair, her hair is layered all the way around her head. She also has face-framing layers to create airy movement and reduce weight in the front. Her hair is then point cut deeper than most people's hair to eliminate bulk. Without layering her hair like this, it takes forever for Caitlin's hair to dry and it hangs very heavy.

Chloe (left) has a great, modified, layered pixie cut! A short length coupled with lots of layers shows off her long neck and brings attention to her eyes and mouth—her faves!

As you can see from the pictures of all these ladies' hairstyles, no matter what kind of hair you have, you can tailor a cut to suit your hair type and texture—as well as your lifestyle—to make the most of what you like best about yourself.

HAUTE COUTURE STYLE *vs.* Fast-Food Beauty

So many women head to the salon hoping—and expecting—to look good when they leave. Instead, many leave feeling like they can't wait for their hair to grow out. That shouldn't be, especially when they are paying hard-earned money for a cut or color to make them look and feel better.

This happens because some stylists follow certain dogmatic "beauty rules" that just don't work for everyone. In this chapter, I explore some of these long-held hair myths and show you why they just don't hold up.

Myth #1:
A Predetermined Face Shape
Determines Your Haircut

This is one of the most pedestrian things I have ever heard from a group of people who refer to themselves as artists. Classifying women's faces in a very rigid way as square, round, rectangular, or whatever is like painting by the numbers.

How many times have you heard someone say, "I can't get that kind of haircut because my face is too round"—or too square? These adjectives suggest something negative about your appearance and limit your options. What a way to start a process that is supposed to make you feel beautiful!

There is a long-held myth that the shape of your face determines the kind of cut you should get. Not so. In my view, the kind of cut I give a woman is all about making her feel and look beautiful, while considering her hair type and texture as well as her lifestyle.

It is my responsibility to be creative and find a way to make what you want work, even if your face is *petite* or *full*, adjectives that I find much more flattering than the harsh geometric rules of thumb that some stylists use to determine how they cut your hair.

I'm not too familiar, however, with the so-called rules about face shapes and haircuts because I never paid much attention to them. To me, these rules are arbitrary. I never understood when someone in beauty school would say, "Oh, Mrs. Reilly is coming in. She has a heart-shaped face, so stick with this cut."

Poor Mrs. Reilly. How long had she and her heart-shaped face worn the same cut? And what if poor Mrs. Reilly's friend Mrs. Fitzpatrick had a long-triangle-square combo? Did she have any options at all?

What if Mrs. Reilly wanted something other than the prescribed cut? My feeling was—and still is—I'm going to give her whatever she wants that will make her feel and look the most beautiful. My job is to interpret what she is looking for and make it modern, relevant, beautiful, and perfect for her. This is what a stylist does. We create *style*.

Today, I hope that young stylists in beauty school look only at the "face" value of the old rules (no pun intended) and appreciate the idea that women do, in fact, have very different face shapes. Most importantly, these rules shouldn't limit their creativity. After all, no two women have exactly the same face shape. To me, these rules create lazy stylists at an early stage in their careers.

Cutting women's hair according to the cookie-cutter face-shape rule is the equivalent of serving customers a meal at a fast-food restaurant: "These are your choices with your burger today. You can have fries and a Coke or fries and a Pepsi." I never wanted to be that type of hairdresser. I'm not into fast-food beauty. My feeling is that as service professionals, we need to do the best job for whoever sits before us in our chairs—and not give them excuses. "Oh, I'm sorry, Mrs. Jones. You have a square face, so you can't have the haircut you want."

I don't like how this fast-food philosophy of beauty is sold to us. It's become a conviction. If you have this skin tone, then you are limited to this. If you are this age, then you can't do that.

I understand the idea behind these rules. But I've never seen them work. It's OK if they're a starting place for stylists to get creative—a stepping-stone to get where they want to go. But the rule can't be their only option.

This is why I subscribe to what I call *haute couture* beauty— custom-tailoring a look for each woman who sits in my chair. You can get an haute couture hairstyle on a budget as long as the cut or look is tailored to your needs—even if you are *square*. You don't have to get a fast-food haircut. Getting an haute couture look has nothing to do with cost. It's a philosophy.

You can get haute couture style by really getting to know your hair, being honest about it, figuring out what you like about it, and asking your stylist for a look that is tailored to you and enhances your favorite features. Being educated will help you get the style and look that's best for you.

What *real women* have to say. . .

"I have had stylists tell me to get a certain cut based on my face shape (not Ken!)," says Helen. *"I have had bad haircuts because of this. Now I just get the cuts I like and they look great—'even' with my round face."*

"I agree with Ken that face shape is irrelevant," says Chloe. *"I have an oblong face shape so according to style guidelines I should not be able to wear my hair short. They are wrong. Short hair suits me perfectly!"*

Myth #2:
The Older You Are, the Shorter Your Hair Should Be

Someone put this big rule out there that when you turn a certain age, you have to cut your hair short. I love short hair. Short hair cut the right way can be very sexy and feminine. But each woman should decide that. No stylist should tell her that's what she *has to do* because she is a certain age. You don't have to have your husband or brother's cut.

I think it's outdated and unliberated to tell women they can't have long hair when they reach a certain age. Rules about hair length and age are silly and antiquated. Women make great decisions for their families, for large corporations, and in world affairs, so why shouldn't they have a say in how they like to wear their hair? Rules like this suggest that someone has power over you to determine how you should look. It makes you want to say, "You're not the boss of me!"

Look at women such as Michelle Pfeiffer, Oprah Winfrey, Demi Moore, Rene Russo, Kim Basinger, and Madonna. They're all in their fifties and have gorgeous, long hair. So do Susan Sarandon, Susan Lucci, Goldie Hawn, Emmy Lou Harris, and Meryl Streep, who are in their sixties, believe it or not.

These women don't follow the rules and they still look amazing, and far younger-looking than they really are. They must be doing something right. I think it has to do with how their hair makes them feel. They are standing for an ideal of beauty, yet we tell the rest of the women in the world what cuts to get at certain ages.

One of the stereotypes I've heard over the years for women in their fifties and beyond is that you should basically get your husband's haircut—supershort and plain. (You could share the same barber!) That to me is unacceptable. (I am all for low maintenance, but I don't think we should ever disregard ourselves. Even wash and wear can look pretty.) According to this stereotype, hair should get progressively shorter as you age. This rule defeminizes women. I don't understand it. It's as if the older you get, the more society wants to take away perhaps the most important thing that we associate with femininity, vitality, and health—your hair.

As I've said before, I am all for what makes you feel beautiful. I love hair that celebrates a woman, whether it is short or long. After all, it is all about you. Be who you are. Wear your hair the way you want to wear it, as long as it's flattering *to you*.

Myth #3:
You Can't Go Blonde
(or Brunette or Red…)

A lot of women tell me they wish they could change their hair color. "Oh, Ken," I hear. "I've always wanted to be a blonde, but I can't." Or "I'd love to go darker, but I can't."

Says who?

You can have any color you want—you just have to make sure the shade or tone complements your skin tone. If you are going for a drastic change, make sure you take the time to do it the right way and keep your hair healthy.

I have made my mother's hair dark brown, medium-brown, and light brown, all the way to very blonde, with and without highlights. We were able to do that because the tone of the colors complemented her olive complexion.

I always love seeing the impact and reaction when I change my clients' hair color, whether by using extensions and hairpieces or coloring their own hair.

I have worked with friends and clients like Eva Longoria, Jennifer Lopez, and Eve, all of whom have naturally dark hair. Throughout the years, I have created looks from dark brown to different shades of blonde for all three women. For them, a change in hair color was all about the moment and how the color matched how each woman wanted to feel. It was the tone that made it their very own. It was under my direction that we took Jessica Simpson from her trademark blonde to the perfect auburn red that was inspired by Norma Jean Baker before she went blonde and became Marilyn Monroe.

Recently on *The X Factor* (USA) stage, I took the first season's competition winner, Melanie Amaro, from a medium brown to a warm chestnut; to a rich, golden honey; then took her to darkest brown; and brought her back to medium brown again. Within the six weeks of live shows we did, we changed Melanie's color countless times, even using hairpieces to go from dark to light and back to dark in one live show. When I met Melanie she had never colored her hair before. Now she is a pro!

If you radically change your hair color, you will get a lot of opinions. And we all know what they say about opinions. But remember, your hairstyle is all about you and what you want.

Finding the Right Hair Color for Your Skin Tone

I'm here to say that you can have whatever color you want, as long as it's the right tone. Just as with interior decorating, fashion, or anything else that has to do with color, you want to choose hues that complement each other.

Your hair is like a frame around your face. We want to make sure that that frame complements your skin. I don't necessarily look at the depth or lightness of skin color when considering hair color. If a woman has the confidence to wear a hair color that is in great contrast to the depth of the color of her skin, the look can be interesting and dynamic, just like the look of a person with dark skin who has light eyes, or a person with very light skin who has very deep, dark eyes—the contrast is exotic and beautiful.

I always look at the undertone in people's skin to choose a complementary tone for their hair. All shades of skin have undertones. The deepest of skin colors can have red, caramel, and olive undertones, as can very light skin. Just like hair textures, your skin tones can also be a combination of several of these colors, so my suggestions are merely a safe starting point:

- If you have red undertones in your skin, I recommend going with a more neutral tone (which does not mean it lacks brightness) or a cool tone for your hair, which will complement the red in your skin and not exaggerate it.

- If you have olive skin, which tends to be on the cooler side and is already somewhat neutral, you can slightly vary the tone in either direction—from cool tones to warmer tones.

You don't want to go too cool with your hair tone, which will appear to draw all the pigment from your skin and make your hair look very ashy. If you go too warm, your hair will look too brassy against the contrast of your cool skin.

Keep in mind that the term "olive skin" suggests a "green" undertone, so anything too ashy (with a green undertone) is too much and anything too warm (with a golden undertone) will be unflattering. There is an area between both which will still give you great variation.

- If your skin has golden or caramel undertones, it's great to stay with neutral warm tones, neutral tones, and neutral cool tones.

- If you have yellow undertones in your skin, warmer tones in your hair will complement your skin. You can have a very neutral caramel complexion and go further into the warmer, golden hair colors.

There are all kinds of variations and combinations of skin tones. I suggest holding sample hair color swatches next to your skin when considering a drastic color change. I have used wigs and extensions on my clients to test a new color before committing to it.

Myth #4:
You Can't Get a Certain Cut Because of Your Hair Texture and Type

Yes, there are even myths about hair texture and type that end up confusing women in the end. I don't think there is only one option for hair textures and types. Beauty as a whole has to be personalized and exceptions to every "rule" have to be made based on each woman's needs, her lifestyle, what her life calls for. You have to feel beautiful just as yourself.

I believe in styles for women that work in real life—styles for women who don't have their hair done professionally every day. You want a style that works with your hair type and texture so you can do it easily—on the go—and still look beautiful, whether you're a busy mom who only has time for a ten-minute beauty regimen wedged in between breakfast and car pooling, or a career woman with a high-pressure job who has just a few minutes to feel put together and polished.

Getting to know your hair by understanding your hair texture and type is a great way to get the right cut for you. Learn to work with it, not against it. A stylist might tell a woman with very curly hair that because of her face shape, she is limited to bangs and a bob. That's great if that's what she wants. But even if you have very curly hair, maybe you don't want bangs and a bob now, let alone for the rest of your life. Be realistic about your hair texture and hair type and go from there. It is what it is. Say it with me: "My hair is fine and it's mine!" You get my drift.

I suggest going to a stylist who is well versed in your hair texture and type and can give you an achievable variety of options based on what you would like from your cut. It's your stylist's job to make what *you* want work for you! Hello, it is all about you!

If you see a woman around town whose hair texture is similar to yours and you like her cut, ask her who cuts her hair. Chances are that stylist will understand your texture and may be able to lead you to the hair of your dreams. It doesn't hurt to have a consultation. It's your hair, so get to know it and understand it—and get what you want.

How to Get the Most Flattering Cut for Your Hair Type and Texture

Understanding your hair type and texture is, in my opinion, the first step to getting a look that works for you. Then you can create a shape that complements your features. I want you to feel beautiful in your own skin…and hair!

It's the stylist's job as an artist to create a look that enhances your unique and individual beauty. The stylist needs to find out what you love about yourself when you look in the mirror and figure out how your hair can enhance that. This look, however, must also work with your hair texture and type as well as your lifestyle. You don't want a cut that requires hours of wasteful time to change your hair texture.

Next, it is important to understand what types of hairstyles appeal to you and understand what it is that you like about that hair. (Pictures are a great reference. Find pictures of hair with texture that is similar to yours.)

More often than not, women like what they don't have. Often a woman with straight hair will say that she loves wavy hair or a woman with curly hair will say she loves a straight style. That has to change.

How Stylists Decode What Women Like and Want

If a woman with straight hair tells me she loves big, voluminous waves, I know it's volume and movement she is after.

If a woman with wavy, curly, or kinky hair tells me she loves sleek, straight hair, I know she is looking to tame and smooth her hair.

This is all very easy to figure out with a few simple questions.

Again, I do believe that a woman with straight hair should have curls when she wants, and vice versa, but I don't think it is realistic or fair to yourself to deny that what you have naturally is beautiful.

Once you've identified what you like about your looks and features and what you would like in a style, your stylist can create a personal look just for you. How refreshing. So different from "No. You can't have that, Miss Square Face…"

It is the stylist's job to help each client understand her hair texture and type. As I've said, the four main hair types are usually kinky, curly, wavy, and straight. Textures are generally coarse, medium, or fine. But guess what? Most people can also have a combination of types and textures. Hair can be curly in the nape, wavy above the ears, and nearly straight on the crown. It's like winning the texture lottery! Lucky you, huh?

Fine, Straight Hair

If you have fine, straight hair and you want texture, volume, and movement, you can create shorter layers, but not too short— no "mall bangs," please! Remember those? Bangs that were sprayed sky-high and stood up straight?

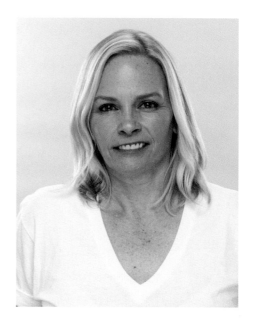

Lisa has a lot of fine hair. The right layers make her hair appear thicker.

If you overlayer straight, fine hair, you'll wind up with even thinner, scragglier ends than when you started. The key is to keep most of the thickness and weight around the base of this cut so it looks voluminous and can support the layers you're creating.

We've all seen women with fine hair whose style collapses or "dents" in under the feathered layers on top. It's almost like she's wearing a triangular hair hat on top of her hair, which leaves you wondering why she doesn't just cut the bottom off. This kind of cut is almost see-through at the bottom. (I hope you're not reading this and thinking, "Oh, no. That's me.")

Very Thick Hair

You can cut into very thick hair to eliminate some bulk and aerate the cut. Keep in mind that coarse hair may become frizzier from thinning shears or razors. My tool of choice for this kind of hair is basic shears.

These basic, classic techniques work for a wide variety of hair types and textures, no matter the length. The length at which you start layering your hair and the extent to which you layer it are the elements that personalize a cut and enhance your features. Once you get to know your hair and how it reacts, you can start experimenting with other techniques.

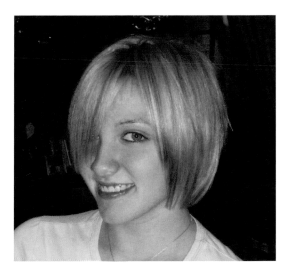

Dont' be afraid to go short. Caitlin's hair is very thick, and we made it work!

Wavy, Curly, or Kinky Hair

If you have wavy, curly, or kinky hair that has a medium or coarse texture and is unmanageable or out of control, proper layering can create a more polished look. Face-framing layers make heavy, overwhelming hair much lighter. But you still need weight on the bottom to pull the hair down and keep it from looking triangular.

A longish, rounded hairstyle is good for hair of this type and texture. Longer, more uniform layers all the way around will eliminate bulk while still looking very current and classic. You can layer—or bevel— the perimeter of this kind of hair so that the edge of your cut is not too heavy or bulky. This type of layering and weight distribution will also work for wavy, curvy, or kinky short styles.

Since I'm usually seen doing hair for women such as Eva Longoria, Victoria Beckham, and Jessica Simpson, who have straight, long hair, a lot of people don't realize that I have styled hair for clients with every hair texture, type, style, cut, and color in the book while doing makeovers on *The Oprah Winfrey Show*, *The Biggest Loser*, *America's Next Top Model*, and *The Doctors*.

I am also proud of my work on the first season of *The X Factor* (USA) for many reasons, but mostly because I was able to celebrate and show the world many different ideals of beauty. One of the contestants I worked with was a beautiful, talented young girl named Rachel Crow, who happened to have the most gorgeous kinky, curly hair. Week after week, I perfected Rachel's curls into a variety of looks that her fans

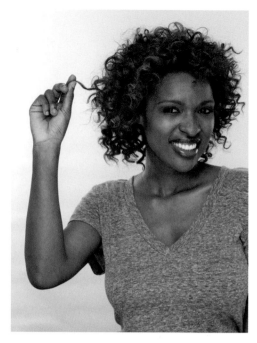

Nyke's layered, face-framing curls

named "The Crow Fro," "The Crow-Hawk," and "Crow Curls."

Often during makeover week on shows like these, kinky curls are straightened. This wasn't the case with Rachel. Kinky conquered! After we did up her 'fro in so many different ways, dozens of women and girls wrote to me and said, "Thank you for celebrating our hair" and "Thank you for showing the world how beautiful our hair is."

In fact, after the show was aired, Dr. Meena Singh, a doctor at the Mayo Clinic in Minneapolis, thanked me for my work with Rachel Crow on the show. Dr. Singh told me that her two young daughters, whose hair is just like Rachel's, never liked their hair and always wanted it straight, like many of their friends, until they saw Rachel Crow performing on *The X Factor* with her big, beautiful, bouncing, kinky curls.

GETTING THE
MOST OUT OF YOUR
Salon Visits

When a woman comes to see me for the first time or when I'm doing a makeover on someone, the first thing I say to her is, "Tell me about you." I need to understand her and find out more about her so I can give her a look that works with her lifestyle. Does she work? What kind of business is she in? Does she stay at home with the kids? What does she do in her day-to-day life?

I also think it's important to set the tone of our meeting with a positive vibe. I try to steer the conversation away from "I hate my hair" or "I don't like..." to something more positive. No Negative Nellies, please. (On a selfish note, I like to make it a positive experience for me, too.)

I find that being positive makes women feel more comfortable and at ease. This definitely helps me when I get to the big question: What do you find most beautiful about yourself? I know that coming to the salon or getting a makeover can be intimidating to begin with, so it is important to me to make a woman feel welcome and relaxed.

Don't Be Afraid of the Woman in the Mirror

Once you were sitting in my chair at the salon, feeling at ease and relaxed, it would be time to address the mirror. This is often the hardest part. I always say, "Let's look in the mirror." If you look at me in the mirror and not yourself, I know I have my work cut out for me. If you look right at yourself, we're ahead of the game.

First, I'd ask you to tell me what you think is beautiful about yourself when you look in the mirror. Sometimes, a client's reaction veers to "Well, I don't like…" But that's not the question. So I'll ask again, "What do you find beautiful about yourself when you look in the mirror?" Chances are that if you don't recognize it now, you will still deny it later. When you can tell me what you love about yourself when you look in the mirror, and truly believe it, I can then enhance it for the rest of the world to see!

Making a Cut Work for You

After the mirror conversation, I also ask, "What is your hair routine?" I like to create a look that is within a woman's capabilities to maintain. There's nothing worse than loving your hair when you leave the salon…until you wash it and are frustrated because it doesn't look at all like it did when you got it done.

Next, we discuss what kind of hair you're attracted to. We look at pictures and flip through magazines. Often a professional stylist's "language" is very different from the client's when you're describing hair. You all know how different an "inch" can be at the salon. The biggest problem preventing you from getting what you want is often a lack of communication or mutual understanding. A picture speaks a thousand words. I say, bring on the pictures. Even though what you like may be unrealistic for your hair type and texture, it helps me understand your taste. It's my job to communicate to you what is feasible.

I also like to ask, "How much time can you commit to upkeep? Do you want to be committed to color? Do you want to be committed to a particular cut?" We'll discuss your hair texture and type, your lifestyle, and how you like to do your hair and the amount of time you have to do it.

If you like a freshly highlighted look with perfect bangs and detailed layers, but only have ten minutes a day to spend on your hair and can get to the salon only twice a year, I may talk you out of that style and into something that requires less commitment. Low mainte-nance does not have to lack style! I'll give you a look that will be easy to style and that will grow out really well, requiring minimal salon visits. Even when I'm doing makeovers, I make sure to give my clients some-thing they'll be able to work with when they're on their own. Women whose hair I've cut and who have waited two years (usually because of my schedule) between cuts have said that their hair has grown out beautifully at every stage of growth.

I take all of this into consideration before I even pick up my scissors.

Communication Is the Key

It's the stylist's job to provide you with an end result that is the perfect combination of your dream hair and what is best and, most importantly, feasible for you. Your relationship is like any other—it takes communication and compromise to be successful. Since you want a look that's beautiful but also realistic, given the time you have every day to maintain it, you need to discuss the following:

- What you find beautiful about yourself when you look in the mirror
- Which haircuts, styles, and colors you are attracted to (bring pictures, if you like)
- Your hair type and texture
- How you normally style your hair
- Your lifestyle
- The amount of time you have to spend on your hair and on maintenance (do you let your hair dry on the way to work after dropping the kids off at school, or do you visit the salon three times a week for touchups and blowouts?)
- Your stylist's experience in working with your hair type and texture
- Based on everything you've said, ask what the stylist envisions for you

While sitting in your stylist's chair, for example, you could say, "I like a lot of the longer hairstyles I see right now that look effortless without a lot of layers." You could show a picture and then ask, "What do you think works with my hair type and texture? I want something I can wear natural and loose on an every-day basis, and I'd like to put no more than fifteen or twenty minutes into it on a normal day." See what your stylist says.

What Should You Look For in a Stylist?

You want to work with a stylist who is willing to listen to you, understands you, treats you like an individual, and is well-versed in your hair texture and type (not every stylist is). Keep in mind that some stylists are better at short hair than longer hair or vice versa. So make sure you find a stylist who works well with the style you're looking for. And if a stylist doesn't listen to you or understand your needs, then it doesn't really matter how talented he is. It doesn't matter if he can cut the straightest line ever—if it's too short and not what you want. Remember—this is about you. It's not about the stylist. You are the consumer paying for a service. (Women tend to forget that sometimes.) You want to leave happy—a haircut isn't a pair of jeans that you can return for a better-fitting pair!

WHEN YOU SEE A STYLIST, *please* go in with an open mind. Remember you pay professionals not only for their service and time, but also for their knowledge and expertise. Express yourself and see how they respond. If you like what they have to say, then stay. If you are uncomfortable with their ideas, then you don't have to stay. Not everyone sees eye to eye. It is better to know this before you start than wait until it's too late.

EARLY ON IN MY CAREER I WORKED AT a place that had an intercom—"Ken, your client is here"—because we were given a time limit for each service. I really hated this system because it let clients I was working with know that their time with me was up, whether my work was finished or not.

We were allowed thirty minutes for a haircut, which included a shampoo, haircut, blow-dry, and styling! Needless to say, I was always running behind, because I *never* agreed with a thirty-minute limit. The salon manager (and I hope she reads this) thought it was a good idea to put a timer on my station and start it at thirty minutes, the moment a client sat down in my chair. All we heard, from the consultation all the way through the cut, was "tick tick tick…" That didn't last. I threw the timer away in front of the salon manager and told her to fire me. She didn't and I continued to give my clients the service they deserved.

Sometimes a Picture Is Worth a Thousand Words

A lot of women tell me that when they go to see a stylist, they find it hard to articulate exactly what it is they want. They might have an idea in mind, but aren't sure how to convey it to the stylist. In these cases, you should bring pictures to use as a reference point and as a way to start a dialogue. You want to be realistic about the outcome, however, so the pictures should show women with the same hair type and texture as yours. This will give your stylist an idea of what you are looking for.

To make sure you get what you are after, it's also a good idea to ask the stylist exactly what she plans to do. Keep in mind, though, that clients and stylists use different words to describe a look. That's where pictures can help your stylist to better understand what kind of look you want. When it comes to color, pictures can also help her understand the color you have in mind for your hair. The fewer surprises, the better.

Once you have settled on a style, be visual about your questions. You may want to ask things like "You're going to cut an inch. Where will that be? How will that bang fall?" Don't let a stylist just start going at your hair with the scissors as soon as you sit in the chair, especially if you are uncertain or still have any unanswered questions. The bottom line here is that the stylist is working for you. You are paying for a service. I have never started cutting a woman's hair without making sure we've spoken and are on the same page. The consultation is essential.

What *real women* have to say...

Helen *says, "A stylist told me that she knew exactly what kind of style I needed for my son, Jon's, wedding to Lisa in 1986. She gave me big curls done with brush rollers. It wasn't combed out. Just hair-sprayed. I went home and shampooed my hair and restyled it myself."*

That's the Color We Talked About?

Communication with your stylist is key to getting the right hair color. You have to be realistic and clear about your hopes for color, but also realistic about what is feasible for your hair. You may want to ask your stylist:

- What do you suggest and why?
- What do you think works with my complexion?
- Can you show me some color swatches or pictures of what you have in mind?
- Will this product damage my hair?
- How much upkeep is there? How fast will the color grow out?

You must also share your hair color (or other chemical) history with your stylist. Color swatches are a great way to visually communicate with your stylist about color. Be sure, when you are looking at swatches, that your stylist understands that you are looking at these colors as "end result" colors—what your hair will look like when it is finished. Often stylists refer to the swatches as the color they will apply to your hair. The way the color "processes" on each person's hair can vary greatly. Be very clear that the color you are looking at and choosing is what you want to see at the end. This way your stylist can adjust your color formula to produce more accurate results. I am also not opposed to looking at pictures to better understand what you want or what you're getting.

If, in your conversations about the color you want, your stylist uses terms such as "warm," "cool," "ash," or any others, ask questions. You should know what you're getting.

Beauty Bullying

When you go to the salon, you expect to come out feeling great. But some stylists focus more on the negatives than the positives, leaving their clients feeling anything but beautiful. This is what I call beauty bullying. I see it all the time—beauty professionals who feel the need to insult what you already have in order to make their work, and what they will do for you, look even better. It's one thing I don't do and don't encourage people in my salons to do, either.

What *real women* have to say...

"A hairstylist in a salon once told me that I have a crazy hairline at the nape of my neck," says Helen. *"And she made sure all the other stylists and staff in the salon knew. I was embarrassed. No matter how well the haircut turned out, all I could think about was how I had an ugly hairline."*

Beauty bullying usually happens when stylists are trying to prove their professional worth to you instead of wowing you with what they can do. When a client says about her current hairdo, "This is really bad, isn't it?" I always reply, "It's not bad. It might not be what I would have done, but that doesn't make it bad." Stylists are artists, and I don't think an artist should judge another artist's work.

10
Fabulous Hair
AT EVERY AGE

I think by now you may have realized that I am not a fan of beauty rules. This is also the case when it comes to looking a certain way—just because you are a particular age. No matter how old you are, you deserve to look current and feel great about yourself.

Embrace who you are *right now*. Let go of what was. Sure, you looked beyond sexy in that frosted Farrah Fawcett cut—in 1977! But we're no longer pulling highlights through a cap...and I hope you're not, either! Now it's time for something fresh.

At the same time, you don't want a look that's completely inappropriate for your age. If you're sixty-five, long platinum extensions might not be the best look for you. If you're in your twenties, you might want to stay away from a nice, safe, plain-Jane "mom" cut.

Bottom line? You want a style that fits your personality, lifestyle, hair type and texture, and that shows off your best features—whether you're 17, 21, 35, 42, 54, 65, or beyond. In this chapter I'll share some tips for great hair at any age that will keep you looking fresh and modern.

If You're in Your Teens and Twenties

This is a great time of self-exploration, personal growth, and risk-taking. (Safe risks, please. Always be smart and trust your gut!) You're figuring out who you are, what you want to do with your life, and what your place is in the world.

You're dating. You're making new friends. You're trying to figure out how you'll support yourself and what kind of career you want. This can be a challenging time. And yes, you will make mistakes along the way, but that's how you learn and evolve into the amazing woman you are becoming.

Again, it all goes back to believing in who you are and doing what you think is right for you. You have the answers. You might not realize it right now, but you do. Trust yourself.

What's so wonderful about this stage of life is that you aren't quite set in your ways yet. This is hopefully a time to explore all the good things that life has to offer and to have some fun. Since there's a lot of self-discovery going on at this age, it's the perfect time for trial and error in your beauty regimen.

What *real women* have to say about...

Their Twenties

"Your twenties is a time that presents you with many opportunities to find yourself," says Caitlin. *"It is a stepping-stone between childhood and the beginning of our adult lives. Many of us think that we know who we are growing up, but we're growing into who we will one day become.*

"College definitely has a major role in sculpting us into who we will be in the future. Throughout these years, we perfect a juggling act between school, work, and a social life. All the built-up stress helps us prioritize our responsibilities while squeezing in time for a personal life. Your twenties are certainly some of the best years of your life and you should live them to the fullest!"

If there's ever a time to be adventurous with your hair, it's when you're in your twenties. While I don't necessarily like to follow trends, I give twenty-somethings a free pass to be "trendy" and experiment with different looks.

Having fun with your outward appearance—hair, makeup, and clothes—is normal and healthy at this age. Trying out different looks allows you to enjoy your beauty and see what works best for you. Doing so will also prevent you from limiting yourself to a certain look, which will help you in years to come.

So try some new things! (It's better to do it now because your hair won't be as forgiving as you get older.) Have fun!

My niece Caitlin, for instance, has already had long, short, red, blonde, and brown hair and pink and purple extensions! (It kind of comes with the territory. I'm her uncle.)

Keep in mind I styled Caitlin's hair once when she was in grade school for "crazy hair" day! She had very long hair. She sat patiently as I curled very small sections with my smallest curling iron. I made sure we had plenty of time before she had to leave for school. I also gave her brother Ethan crazy hair that day—a blue Mohawk.

After her hair was all curled, I teased it to the sky! She was four foot nine and tiny as can be. Her hair was two feet wide and one foot tall! It was crazy, all right. When it was time for school, Ethan went to catch the bus and Caitlin caught one look at herself in a mirror and burst into tears!

Hey, I was already a "celebrity hairstylist" and this was definitely crazy hair! I was devastated that my princess was in tears! She missed the bus and was late for school. I did everything I could to make her feel better, but that hair wasn't going anywhere. It was teased and sprayed to the max.

I managed to make it look smaller, enough to convince Caitlin to let me drive her to school. Class was well under way when we arrived. Caitlin began to wail again. I felt horrible. We finally got out of the car and walked into the office to explain what happened. All the while, Caitlin still had tears in her eyes and was saying, "Uncle Kenney, I really don't want to go." As soon as I got her signed in, another student walked by and said, "Wow, Caitlin, cool hair!" She stopped crying immediately and took off. From a distance I heard a happier "Bye, Uncle Kenney!"

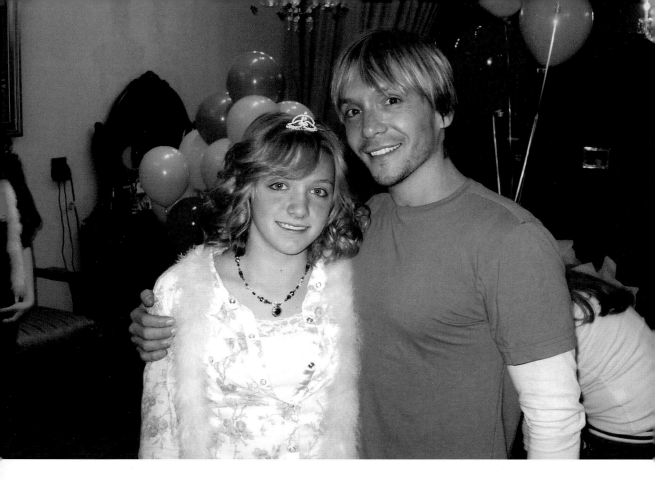

This was certainly not the last time Caitlin would have a radical hair change. When Caitlin turned thirteen, I staged a makeover birthday party at the salon for her and thirteen friends. They all got whatever they wanted—with their parents' approval: a cut, color, purple or pink extensions, makeup. The works.

Just for fun I had all the girls take turns with my scissors, cutting Caitlin's hair as I supervised. Then all the girls colored her hair too! It was so much fun. Imagine how hard you laugh with thirteen 13-year-old girls cutting and coloring their friend's hair! Caitlin was a good sport and I made sure her hair looked great!

When Caitlin was a little older, she modeled various hair products for me. I was always doing something to Caitlin's hair. When she was fifteen, she and her family came to visit me in Los Angeles. We gave her permanent extensions (she had only worn clip-ins before). We went to Disneyland and I told everyone else in all the lines, "Caitlin's wearing a weave!"

I don't know if Caitlin or I have had more fun changing her hair over the years. I do know that because Caitlin has had so many different looks she does not define her beauty by her hair or any particular style. Caitlin has superthick hair, which could actually reach her waist if she let it grow. She has worn her hair very long in the past but now it's shorter. I'm sure it will change the next time I get my hands on it! After all, she is only twenty!

I say anything goes when you're in your twenties—long or short, modern or classic, light or dark, straight or curly, and anything in between. Figure out now what works for you and definitely what doesn't! I have known Nyke for two years now and we have already changed her hair many times. Long and dark, short and curly, with extensions, without extensions and natural, wavy and auburn, bangs and no bangs, highlights and no lights! Every one of those styles looked great.

If You're in Your Thirties

Wow, are you busy! You've most likely chosen a career path and are working hard to get ahead, which can mean long days and nights at your workplace. If you're married or in a relationship, you have to squeeze in a little quality time with your significant other and/or family. Or you might be just starting a family, which means nonstop diaper changes, round-the-clock feedings, and little time—if any—for you. With all you have to do and all you're accountable for, you're probably not as carefree as you used to be. You have more responsibilities now—including the responsibility you may feel now to look "responsible," "serious," or "grown up."

In my thirties, I remember wanting to look "mature" so that people would take me seriously as a beauty expert. It wasn't until I was almost forty that I stopped wearing a suit or a sport coat every time I appeared on television. Now I don't want to look "stuffy" or too "serious."

When it comes to your hair, though, being "grown up" and "serious" doesn't have to mean mediocre, boring, or looking like everyone else. You can be taken just as seriously with a style that's beyond flattering—whether it's long, short, or somewhere in between. Why? Because you want to show the world what a radiant, strong, confident, capable, and yes, flirtatious, fun woman you are. You are in your thirties! You are young and vibrant. You are definitely sexy. And you look fantastic! Show how great you feel with a versatile, sexy cut.

So many women tell me that they want to chop off their hair at this stage of their lives to make it easier to style. They like being able to just wash it and go. One woman said to me, "Ken, I have three little kids—a four-year-old, a two-year-old, and a three-month-old baby. Are you kidding?! I have no time to do anything with my hair."

I get it.

While I do love short hair, a plain-Jane "mom" cut doesn't have to be in your future. A "sexy mom" cut? I'm OK with that.

With all you have going on in your life, *don't forget yourself.* You are still your own woman. Your hair should communicate exactly how you *really* feel, deep down. Maybe it's "I am still beautiful, even though I get home from work at ten most nights" or "I still feel sexy deep down, even though I have spit-up on my shirt."

The difference is that you know more now than you did when you were younger, and you are getting a better handle on things. I like to think you're becoming more polished—and your hair should reflect that—even if it's not the case. Looks can be deceiving, sometimes in the best possible way. Why not look "together," even if you're not? Maybe you'll start believing it yourself.

What *real women* have to say about...

Their Thirties

"I love my thirties," says Sarah M. *"They've been the most productive and best years of my life. In your twenties you're still figuring out what you want to do with your life. You get married and have kids. I'm actually excited about my forties, too. Being forty is like being in your thirties now. I have girlfriends in their fifties who look absolutely amazing. It's all about how you feel inside. It's all about your mind-set."*

As I've said before, to me there are no rules. If short hair makes you feel like a million bucks, then get a short, sexy cut. The same goes for long hair and shoulder-length hair. Remember, fabulous ladies—we are starting a beauty revolution here! I want you to look and *feel* your best, no matter how chaotic your life might seem right now.

I have worked with my very good friend Victoria Beckham, who is in her thirties, to style her very sexy and sophisticated short hair, as well as her effortlessly chic longer locks. Each style was just as beautiful in the moment.

This is a time to evolve your look from whatever you had when you were in your twenties. Now that you're in your thirties, understanding your hair texture and type will save you a lot of time and give you the polished yet sexy, versatile look you deserve.

You can still get it all done and still look great doing it. I promise!

Sarah Magness is a busy wife and mother of two. When I say busy, I mean busy. I don't know how she does it all and still manages to look impeccable at all times. Sarah also owns her own clothing lifestyle brand, "So Low." Sarah's career has evolved in her thirties, so she is now producing and directing movies. Somehow, she also finds time to stay fit, exercising regularly and doing yoga.

Sarah has had short blonde hair, long blonde hair, wavy hair, and straight hair. Sarah's hair is now a rich and luxurious red that she mostly wears straight. This gives her a polished, professional look, but the versatile face framing and long layers of her hair give Sarah the option of many hairstyles, including my trademark waves, which she loves. Whatever she is wearing, however her hair is styled, Sarah radiates class and elegance and an inner confidence that I wish I had.

My good friend Tip, who is in her thirties, is now a successful hair-stylist. Although she loves her natural, tousled, beach waves, we have updated her look. Still effortless, her style too is more polished. Tip knows how important the health of her hair is to the overall look. Her glamorous beach waves don't look like they've spent too much time in the sun. Keeping her hair hydrated and conditioned keeps the quality of her hair looking luxe, like the hair of an accomplished woman in her thirties. Her long, rounded layers are versatile enough to smooth out into sleeker styles, as well.

If You're in Your Forties

You are in your prime. Let's face it. Whether you think so or not, you look great. You're a goddess. With your teens, twenties, and thirties behind you, you've come into your own. You know who you are. You are attractive, sexy, and confident. You don't care what people have to say about you or to you at this point. When life's challenges come at you, you handle them just fine, thank you very much. Whether you believe it or not, all this is true. You have had enough life experiences to know who you are and you should be confident enough to believe in yourself! Own it! I know—I'm forty-one now myself, and I own it!

At the same time, this is an age when many women start bemoaning the fact that they're getting older. They might start seeing some wrinkles or noticing that they don't have the same level of energy they had in their twenties and thirties. Some women embrace this age as one of the best of their lives. Others focus on the negatives.

What *real women* have to say about...

Their Forties

"I feel confidant in who I am as a woman, wife, and mother," says Lisa, *who is forty-seven. "I no longer guess if I'm doing things right. I know my actions and decisions are right for me and I feel I have found myself. I finally get who I am and love who I've become. I know I will never stop growing and changing throughout my lifetime and that is what makes life exciting. I embrace new experiences and look for them now."*

When it comes to hair, I find that many women in their forties resort to getting a haircut like their mothers have. That's not a bad thing, but you don't have to get your mom's haircut now, if ever. Today's forty is not yesterday's forty. If you like this style, then opt for an updated, modern bob that still has flair, or go for a short layered cut that has more sass than you know what to do with! The point is whatever cut you choose should make you feel beautiful, like a million bucks, and anything but average. Remember, you are you, one of a kind. Exquisite and unique. (If you don't talk about yourself like that, you'd better start!)

Today, a woman in her forties owns her looks and makes no apologies for who she is. She loves who she is. (If you still don't, keep reading.)

You don't have to go shorter or lighter, for that matter, according to the old rule. (By now, you know how I feel about "rules.") But if you want to, make it rock! Come on, it's OK to turn heads in your forties!

This is a time, however, to avoid doing anything too severe with your hair or your looks. I always tell my clients that you don't want anything that's too long, too short, too dark, too light, or too anything. Believe it or not, this is when a more natural look will really begin to enhance your beauty.

This is an age when you definitely want to look effortless—like you're not trying too hard. You will certainly be flattered when you hear your friends ask, "How does she do it?" In fact, your entire beauty regimen should become effortless. With everything you are learning about yourself from this book, it will be. Work with what you've got. Stop fighting how beautiful you are!

Charlene, in her early forties, loves her curly hair. Many women in their forties with tight curly hair feel the need to smooth it out because they believe it will look more sophisticated that way. Do not deny your natural sophistication! Charlene is one of the chicest women I know. We have traveled the world together, and from fashion shows in Paris to long hours as a fashion stylist on set, Charlene's style never misses a beat. Her best accessory is her fabulous curly hair.

When you love it, you can flaunt it, and that's OK. Charlene's curly hair is layered to create movement, and she keeps it at a length that gives her volume. Keeping her curls well conditioned, she also has the versatility of blowing her hair straight when she wants to.

My sister-in-law Lisa is always on the go. She represents many of you ladies out there who dedicated much of their thirties and forties to raising their children. Lisa and my brother Jon encouraged all their children to try sports, music, drama, group camping trips, and other activities to help their kids flourish and find themselves. This meant a full-time calendar for Lisa, juggling everyone's agendas, often leaving little time for herself. Over the last few years Lisa has really learned to work with her hair. She was always naturally very blonde, a color that looks great on her. She did manage to find time to keep her hair color up (at the Ken Paves Salon that my mom and dad run in Michigan) as well as growing out her hair to the longest it had been in years. Lisa has a lot of fine hair and discovered that with the right layers she can grow it to a great length that offers her a lot of easy styling options.

What I am about to tell you is exactly why I am writing this book. While Lisa's hair was looking great, and she loved the versatility—I'm always saying it is all about living in the moment! When Lisa was in Los Angeles with my mom, Caitlin, and Chloe (Lisa's youngest child, and my mini-me look-alike) for the photo shoot for this book, she got in the moment! I asked Lisa and Caitlin if either of them wanted to change their hair at all, to try a new cut for the book. They each said no, they were really happy with what they had. I asked if Lisa was open to my cutting a short wig on her just to show how different looks can work. She said sure, since she had worn her hair short years ago.

The next day, she tried on the wig and I gave it a short, modern, sassy, and cool cut. Lisa's eyes lit up! We had already done some amazing pictures with her long hair, but now in this moment, she was loving it short! It looked amazing and made her feel like a million bucks. Although she had felt beautiful every step of the way, you could see this short cut just had to be! She loved the shorter look so much that she had her hair cut short when she got home, at my salon in Michigan. The bottom line: Get to know your hair and what your options are—you should be confident enough now in your forties to live in the moment. It's a beautiful place to be.

For women in their forties, I like classic looks with personality and movement, to keep things chic and sexy. Who doesn't want to be called chic and sexy in their forties?

If You're in Your Fifties, Sixties, and Beyond

You are wise. You should be your most confident and more content than you've ever been in your life. You're nobody's fool. Younger generations come to you for advice because you most certainly know who you are. If not, let me help!

If you have children, they may be almost out of the house, or grown with families of their own. You may be thinking of retiring.

Just like your forty-something sisters, though, you might be feeling your age a lot more these days. You might have aches and pains that weren't there before. You might wonder where the time went. All the more reason not to give up and look defeated. You deserve to look and feel beautiful.

Some women this age decide—this is my time. They want a look that's playful and flirtatious, to celebrate the strong women they've become and the freedoms they now enjoy, now that they're done raising children or are finishing their career. Many others, though, opt for "safe" cuts. They feel that since they're getting older, they have to look more staid and reserved, which can border on boring. Earlier, I pointed out how many women in their fifties, sixties, and seventies start getting cuts that look just like their husband's. STOP the nonsense! Your husband married you, not himself!

Husband Haircut Confidential

I know I've told you ladies *never* to get your husband's cut. But I have a confession: I gave my mom a man's haircut to pass my state board cosmetology test when I was on my way to becoming a professional stylist.

I brought my mom with me to the state board exam to be my model. One of the tasks was to give our models a haircut. I snipped away and finished really early. Mom and I looked around the room and saw that everyone else was still cutting. So she said, "Kenney, keep cutting!" So I kept cutting. At that time I only knew how to do four haircuts. I had already given Mom the first cut I knew, so I now gave her the second one I knew. I finished that one pretty quickly too. Everyone else was still cutting, so she said, "Keep going." So I gave her the third cut I knew.

When I finished with that cut, we saw that everyone else was still busy cutting. Mom repeated, "Just keep going!" I tried to whisper why I shouldn't, but we weren't supposed to be talking. She shhh'ed me and mumbled, "Keep cutting." I wanted to pass the test so I gave her the fourth and final cut I knew—a short, man's haircut.

I finished now with all the other students. There were no mirrors for my mom to see the end result of all that cutting. Before we left, she stopped off to use the bathroom. On her way in, I said nervously, "I'll wait out here with Dad." She came out of the bathroom and said, "I told you to keep cutting." What a great sport! We laughed the whole way home.

I passed the exam. (Thanks, Mom!) And that, my friends, was the last time I ever gave a woman "her husband's cut."

Accept It: You've Still Got It!

I think it is particularly important at this time in your life for you to be the one who reminds the world (and yourself) that you've still got it!

Practically speaking, though, I do believe that a woman in her fifties (and beyond) doesn't want to spend a long time doing her hair every day. She doesn't want to work so hard to feel beautiful. She's absolutely right.

The reason so many women wind up with basic, short haircuts that make them look ordinary is because they're easy to style and maintain. I understand that. Women at this age want to enjoy life more. They don't want to waste time "getting ready." They think, "Been there, done that, got other things to do."

I agree to a degree. I don't think you should spend hours getting ready, but I do think it's healthy not to forget yourself. It is very important to me that the reason is, truly, that you don't want to waste time getting ready and not that you don't want to look in the mirror. I know things may be changing, but you are still beautiful! Take the time, even a few minutes a day, to greet yourself, look yourself in the eye, say "Hi," accept yourself, and, beyond that, honor yourself.

I hope by this point in your life you have realized how unique you are and stopped comparing yourself to everyone else's standards.

Now, let's keep you sassy and classy in your fifties, sixties, and beyond. And dare I say it? Even sexy! The dictionary defines sexy as "generally attractive or interesting." Every woman should feel attractive and interesting at every age. If you feel this way about yourself, so will everyone else.

Looking great is a frame of mind and all women possess the ability to project an image to the world that says "I am beautiful." It's the result of embracing and loving your life, enjoying a good laugh as often as possible, being grateful for the people in your life and all that you have, looking at the bright side of things, being proud of who you are, and

Helen, at 58, looking glamorous and sexy with a long, cool fringe

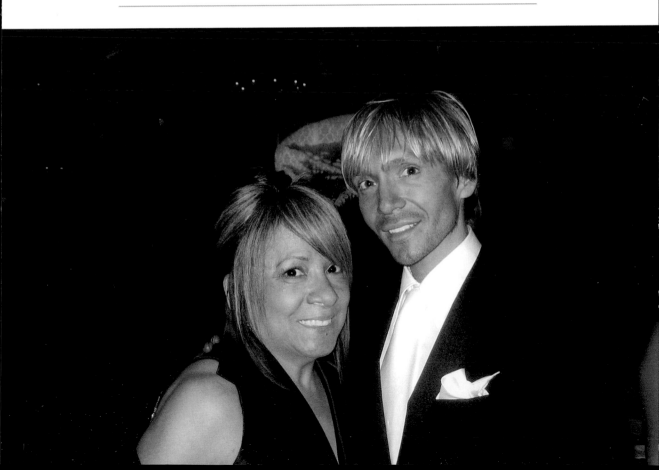

taking time out to acknowledge yourself. Sometimes my job is to give people a reason to look in the mirror and like what they see! There is nothing wrong with that.

When my mom turned sixty, I wanted to do something special for her. I decided to take her to Las Vegas to see Celine Dion's *A New Day* and meet Celine. I was working with Celine and had designed all the hair for the show. I wanted my mom to be present in the moment. I wanted her to look in the mirror and love the image she saw looking back at her. So before we left I gave her a sexy shorter cut with a long cool fringe, similar to the cut Victoria Beckham would later have, and which everyone loved. To make it even more exciting, I gave her very blonde highlights. She loved the cut and felt great about herself. She felt brand-new. That's what this is all about: feeling great about yourself and facing life with a positive attitude. How you look definitely influences how you feel.

Now in her late sixties, my mom is the perfect example of a woman who honestly accepts her beautiful self. She is not disillusioned about what she looks like, she isn't trying to be anyone else, and she's not even trying to look the way she used to look. Helen's secret to being her most beautiful self comes from within. She loves to laugh. She loves to have fun. She is engaged in life and she loves who she is. She is living in the moment.

No matter how old you are, having a fun, positive outlook on life and feeling good about yourself—and who you are as a person—will make you feel alive!

What *real women* have to say about . . .

Fifty

"This is a great decade for me," says Chloe, *who's fifty-four. "Not to say that life doesn't have its ebb and flow, but I have enough of a foundation to know that when it's ebbing, it's going to be OK. I have a little more patience now and I try to live moment to moment, day to day. I'm much more of a spiritual person now, too.*

"In my twenties I was a very rebellious person. I was very hard. My look was androgynous and severe. Think Grace Jones.

"In my thirties I became softer and my femininity blossomed. I met my first husband and we had a son. In my forties I was divorced and focusing on raising my son. I met my second husband in my mid-forties. I would say the end of my forties was fantastic, but my fifties have been the best. I'm just having a blast and looking forward to my sixties!"

Being Over Sixty

"I love where I'm in my life right now," says Helen, *who is sixty-eight. "People say age is just a number, but when you get into your sixties, age is a reality. Everywhere I have been and everything I have done, my family, my friends, and myself—sixty-eight years' worth and it's all mine! Because I have accepted the way I look at this age, I feel more content and satisfied with my life. I love my hair, because the cut and color is what I want. It makes me feel so good when people compliment my hair. For years I tried to keep up with the trends, and with Ken's help, I had every cut and color.*

"Since I was in my fifties, I realized the haircut that makes me happy and looks good on me is the bob in one form or another. I feel it works for anyone at any age. I have had so many variations and it always looks new. I still have some issues with certain body parts, but have learned to work with them and love what God has given me. I used to think about surgery to change things, but now I'm glad. I may not always be thrilled with the way I look at times, but I do love myself and my life in my sixties. I feel pretty, witty, and definitely wise!"

All About Afton

Afton Blake, who is in her sixties now, has been a loving part of my life for more than ten years. She is very positive and radiates love. She has always been there for me and encouraged me to believe in myself and to serve a greater purpose than just me.

Afton, much like Tip, floats around in a bubble of positive energy that she shares with everyone around her. Everything Afton wears means something to her—it is from a special friend or a special place. It may not be the trendiest of fashions, but she always looks beautiful! Afton reminds me of Mother Earth.

For years Afton wore her silvery gray hair very long and always pulled back. I am proud to say that Afton is a cancer survivor. After she lost her hair to cancer, she kept it short for years. I would give her great little choppy cuts all the time. Recently, Afton decided to work on her outside, physical body, since she is always working on her spirit. As a result, she has lost a considerable amount of weight.

Now Afton has decided to grow her beautiful gray hair long again, and I support her. It makes her feel beautiful in this moment, and that looks beautiful to me! Afton loves movement in her hair, so she has a modern shag with tons of layers and a heavy fringe. It is "wash and go," and she loves it.

Beauty is not about trying to recapture your youth. It's about living in the moment and loving who you are. There are so many great moments ahead—don't waste them by not recognizing how beautiful you are today.

I am not saying that liking what you see in the mirror will make your life perfect. No. You will still have challenges; you'll still have both good times and bad. Sometimes the chaos of life can lead us to neglect ourselves. Sometimes we don't want to see ourselves, sometimes we'd rather not look, and sometimes we just don't care. You may not always feel like it, but you are the center of your own life and you have to start putting yourself first…OK, at least considering yourself. That starts by looking in the mirror when you get out of the shower or bath with wet hair and saying, "Hey, good-looking!"—and believing it.

11

ALL
ABOUT...
Ease

A big part of feeling good about yourself is looking your best whenever you can. That's not always easy when you're juggling kids, work, friends, husbands, boyfriends, or the drama du jour.

Whether you're racing out the door on Saturday morning to run errands or tired of fighting with your hair every morning before work, here are some beautiful, everyday looks for those times when you are on the go. After all, you want to make the most of that beautiful canvas you have to work with.

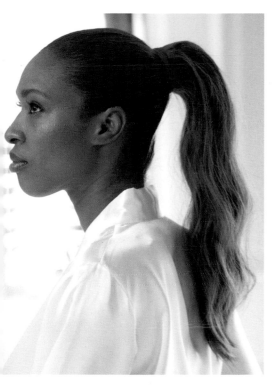

The Essential Ponytail

Ponytails are fantastic when you're pressed for time. But you need to choose the right ponytail if you want to look put-together. A lot of women like to wrap an elastic band low or almost near the bottom of their ponytails. I don't understand this. It looks sloppy, like you've been running around all day and your ponytail is slipping. Saggy and baggy ponytails are not flattering to anyone.

There is a difference between a ponytail that looks fun, fresh, and effortlessly chic, and one that looks like you've been spring cleaning. The right ponytail can take you from running errands to a night out with friends or right onto the red carpet.

Whether it's a high, medium, or low ponytail, too much slack in the back isn't good for anyone. I am all about effortless, simple hair. When pulling your hair into a high pony, sweep it up—back and away

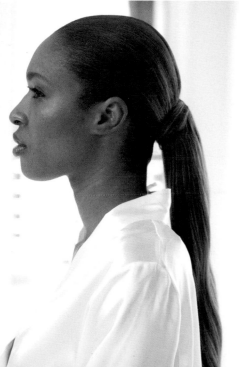

TOP: A high ponytail can give you an instant facelift.
BOTTOM: A low ponytail, tight in the nape—instant chic!

from your face—and secure it in place with an elastic band around your hair slightly back from your crown or even a little lower toward the back of the head. The hair pulling up and away from your face can create a youthful or dramatic appearance. Jennifer Lopez taught me how to do a really good ponytail. She jokingly told me, "If we lose the shape, we lose the game!" It is all about the shape.

Medium and low ponytails are always classic. A low ponytail secured tightly at the nape of your neck can give you a clean, classic, and demure look. It is understated yet makes a statement.

Headbands, Ribbons, and Scarves

Headbands are classic. They never go out of style. Even short-haired women can wear headbands. My friend Victoria Beckham is the perfect example of someone who knows how to wear headbands. She has

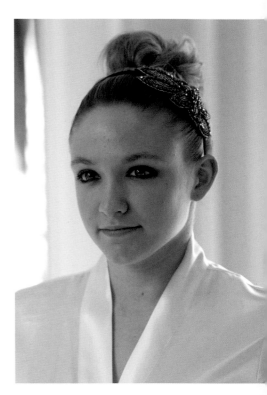

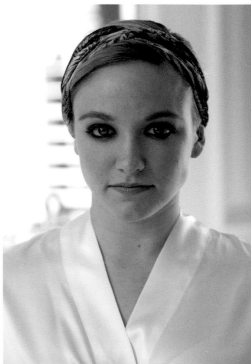

Whether your hair is acting up or you want to give your look a little something extra, a headband, a headband scarf, or even ribbon from the fabric store can be a chic, pretty, and fresh way to give your hairstyle a new attitude.

worn them with short hair, worn them with longer locks for a cool, edgy vibe, aimed for the sweet, demure *Breakfast at Tiffany's* look, and even tried very sleek, mod styles. She's worn everything from leather and lace to metal and flowers! Whether simple or eccentric, I love the detail that a headband can add to your look.

Use a headband to pull all your hair off your face for a clean look or create a more interesting look by working it into your style.

Another way to add polish to your look in seconds is to use a band of fabric or ribbon (a seventy-five-cent purchase that can change your whole look). You can tuck it away under

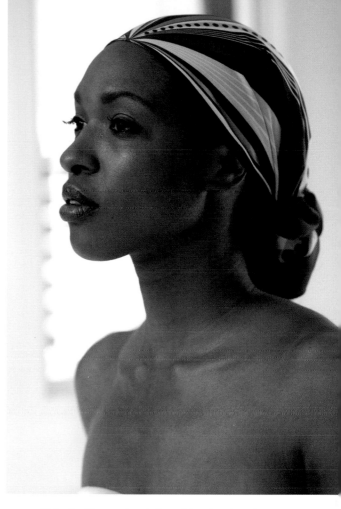

Nyke, looking cool and elegant in a headscarf

your hair or let it hang loose. My one rule about headbands, ribbons, or any hair accessory: Don't wear anything that looks like it belongs on a toddler or a pet.

Another essential accessory is the scarf. Women like Jackie O and Ali MacGraw made wearing headscarves überchic. This is one of my favorite looks of all time. There is no such thing as a bad hair day when you have a great scarf!

Tying a headscarf

Begin by centering the scarf or wrap on your head. Pull down each side evenly. Cross each side over and under your hair. Tie the two ends over the back of the scarf. Braid or twist your hair with the two ends of the scarf and then fold into itself to secure. Voilà! You are ready for the French Riviera or a quick trip to the mall.

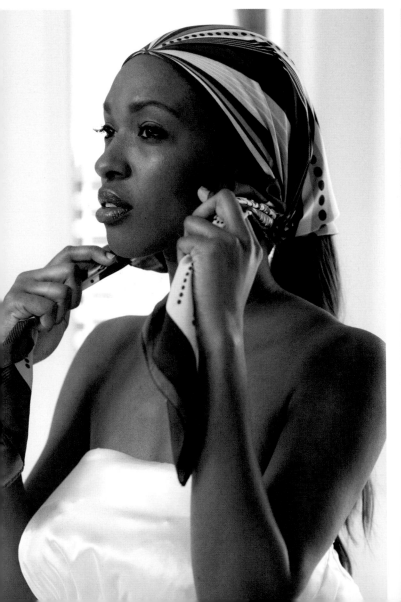
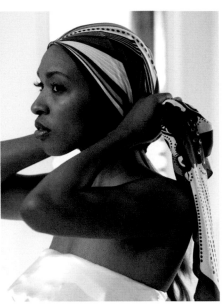
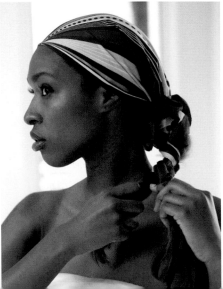

Hair Tricks to Save Time in the Morning

Not shampooing your hair every day will keep it healthier. But as we all know, second-day hair doesn't always look as good as hair does after a fresh wash and style. I'm happy to say that second-day hair never has to look so-so.

How to Use a Volumizer Without Creating Cotton Candy Hair

You can refresh thin, fine hair in seconds by spraying on a volumizer to energize lifeless locks. Different than a dry shampoo, a volumizer adds just enough moisture to dry hair to get rid of bumps and lumps from lying on a pillow all night. You can either finger-style to fluff up your hair or use a blow-dryer and brush just at your roots for extra oomph!

First, here's what to avoid: Don't bend over and spritz away at the ends of your hair with volumizer. When you flip your head back up, the ends of your hair are matted together and look like cotton candy.

Volumizers are intended to give you volume where you need it the most, at the roots. When using a volumizer, focus on the roots—not on the hair that everybody sees. You spray at the root because this is where your hair's natural oils are, where your hair is the healthiest and the heaviest. The spray gives you stiffness and hold; the alcohol in the product dries the oil at the roots, giving you the volume you're seeking.

Start wherever you part your hair. Take a section of hair that's a half-inch to an inch on either side of or behind your crown, lift that section up, and spray into the roots from behind the section. You want to create volume and texture in the interior of your hair and keep the top layer that you see smooth. Keep going until you reach the hair at the nape of the neck. I promise you your hair will definitely stand at attention! Finger-style it for a more natural, tousled look.

Note: Volumizers are usually intended for use on damp, not dry hair. To use a volumizer on damp hair, follow the same directions (above) for sectioning and product application.

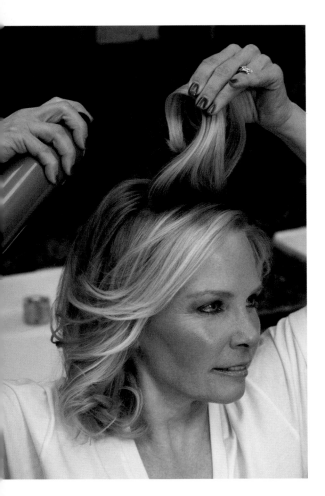

The Right Way to Apply a Finishing or Shine Serum

If you have curly, wavy, coarse, or kinky hair, you can use a shine serum to smooth out any frizz. This will even work on flat ironed or straight hair.

Women tell me that when they apply a finishing product like shine serum to their hair, it looks greasy—especially on the second day. That's because many women start by putting serum in their hands, then wiping it across the top of their heads. Yep, that will have you looking greasy in no time. Most of the product winds up right on the top of your head, on the top layer of your hair, instead of where you really need it.

Spray the volumizer at your roots to give your hair volume where you need it most.

Applying the product the right way will keep your hair from looking greasy:

- Put the product on the palms of your hands, and then rub your palms together to evenly distribute the product. Everyone's hair is different, so apply the serum only where you need it, usually from the midshaft to the ends.

- Take two-inch sections on each side of your head starting at the bottom and "swipe" on top of and under your hair, holding each section between your palms, like you would use a flat iron (see photo).

- Don't press too hard; you want to save some product for the other sections of your hair. When you are finished with both sides, you can use whatever product is left on your hands to spot treat areas that may need more.

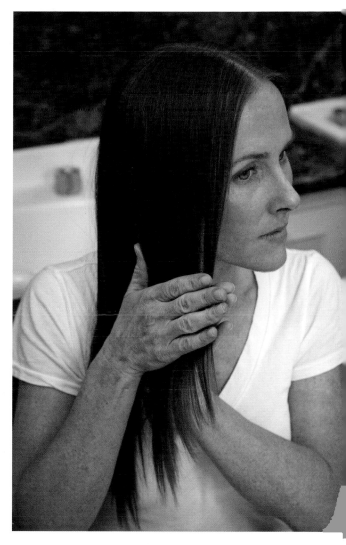

The best way to evenly distribute hair product—with the palms of your hands.

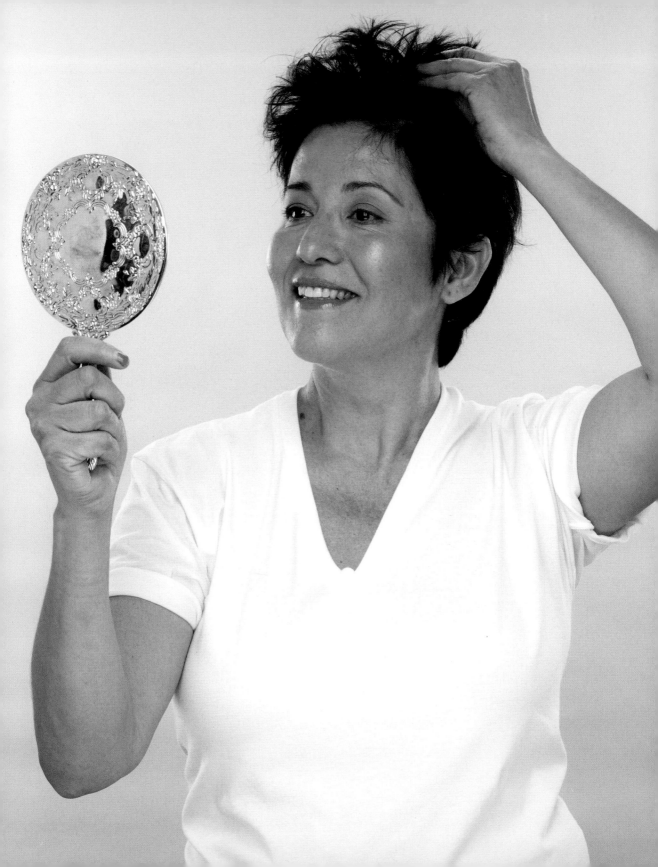

Short-Hair Chic

If you have short hair, it can look matted and messy on the second day after a shampoo. Sometimes all you need is a light spritz of water and some finger-styling to freshen up your short cut. If your hair needs a little more help, you can redefine your style with a small amount of gel. For a softer look, you can mix a little shine serum into your gel. Gel on dry hair seals the cuticle, defines your style, gives you hold, and adds extra shine. A little goes a long way.

Second-Day Hair Saves

- **If you have a textured cut:** Go through your hair with a gel and simply finger-style it back into place.

- **If you have a sleek, straight style:** Use a hair crème, a light pomade, or a shine serum to smooth the hair and give it a hydrated, more finished look.

- **For any kind of hair:** If you have flyaways on top of your head and down the length of your hair, smooth it at the top with a small amount of shine serum or even hand lotion. Avoid too much hairspray on top or you could end up looking "wiggy" instead of *au naturel*. I don't even like my wigs to look "wiggy"!

- **The switcheroo:** Another quick way to give yourself a fresh look is by parting your hair differently than you normally do. Flip your hair to the other side of your head when styling it in the morning. This will give your hair more body within seconds.

12

GLAMOUR GIRL
HAIR...
Va-Va-Voom!

Every woman deserves to have her own red carpet moments, whether it's for a night out with that special someone, a good friend's wedding, a rocking New Year's Eve party, or a trip to the mall with the girls, and you just want to feel fab!

In this chapter I'll show you how to create truly glamorous hair. Glamorous doesn't mean over-the-top or outrageous. It's just a reason for you to strut your stuff!

This is Hollywood hair with tons of sex appeal—hair that is attention-getting and empowering and makes you feel like you are every inch a woman—hair that women dream of having and men dream of their women having. It's sexy even when you're cooking dinner. I guarantee that you will look and feel the most glamorous you've ever been in your life after following the tips in this chapter.

Every woman has an inner lioness. Hair like this lets that lioness come out. It lets her purr.

Glamorous hair can be teased and twisted or tousled and wind-blown; it can be big and voluminous with texture that moves, sleek-shiny and straight, swept up in a sensuous chignon, or an Old Hollywood style. No matter which way you wear it, glamorous hair embraces your feminine power. Now you know you're glamorous. Let's go!

What *real women* have to say about . . .

Looking and Feeling Glamorous

"When I want to get glamorous, 99.9 percent of the time I go for something easy because I'm always in a hurry," says Sarah M. *"But I do like to get glammed up. I think most women do. It's fun. When you lose your desire to be glamorous, I think you've lost your mojo. As a mother and businessperson, I know it's easy to get bogged down by all the stuff in your life. But you have to still stay fresh, look good, and look sexy. It keeps you feeling alive."*

Curl Power!

Whether your hair is long, short, or in between, a few minutes with a curling iron can make your hair look like you spent hours on it when you didn't. You can use a curling iron to enhance your natural curls or waves or give your straight or wavy hair more bounce.

Curling Iron 101

Prepare Your Hair

As with a flat iron, make sure your hair is dry before using a curling iron. I always begin with a thermal protective spray. If you're touching up your wavy or curly hair, you may want to apply some shine serum from the midshaft down. Naturally wavy or curly hair tends to be coarse, so this will help hydrate your style and keep it from getting frizzy. Allow the serum to penetrate and be absorbed by your hair before you begin to use a curling iron. You don't want to fry your hair.

Choose the Right Iron

First, decide what you're looking for—a loose bend or bump, cascading waves, or a natural-looking tight curl. Then choose your curling-iron size accordingly.

Contrary to what you might think, the larger the barrel, the less curl you get. Large barrels produce loose curls and smaller barrels will give you tighter curls. A two-inch barrel will give your hair a slight wave and a bend, rather than a real curl. (In the 1950s and '60s, women would wrap their hair around tin cans and toilet paper rolls to straighten their hair and give it the bubble bouffant look that was all the rage back then.)

My go-to curling iron of choice—the one that offers me the most versatility—is a one-inch barrel. I use many other sizes as well, but I can achieve a soft wave or uniform curl with a one-inch iron.

Also, pick a curling iron that feels comfortable in your hand and is easy to maneuver. Getting the right feel for using the curling iron can take a few tries if you've never used one before.

How Much Heat to Use

Most curling irons have variable settings. The amount of heat your hair needs to achieve a curl varies as much as the settings. The general rule is that fine hair needs less heat, medium hair needs slightly more, and coarse hair needs the most heat. This doesn't always mean using the highest setting. Your goal is to keep your hair healthy. So I don't recommend curling your hair every day and I definitely don't recommend singeing it into submission. I suggest beginning at a low heat at first.

> Curl your ends last, and briefly, since they tend to be the driest part of your hair.
> Using flat irons and curling irons is a luxury afforded to those who have worked hard to keep their hair healthy.

Après Cool-Down Styling

Fight the urge to touch your hair after you curl it. Allowing it to cool before you style it will help lock the curl in place.

After your curls have cooled, you can style them into place. Most often I finger-style curly looks, using a little shine serum. Brushing out curls is usually for looser sets or for vintage or Old Hollywood looks. This creates a very fluffy, pillowing style. For very tight natural sets, I separate and stretch the curls individually with my hands, using either a glosser or light shine pomade to hydrate and seal the ends.

Hair That Doesn't Hold a Curl

If, however, your hair doesn't hold a curl well or if you need your style to last, set it in place before it cools. After you remove each section of hair from the iron, while it's still warm, pin the curl in place with a bobby pin

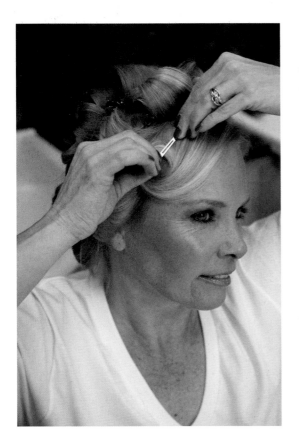
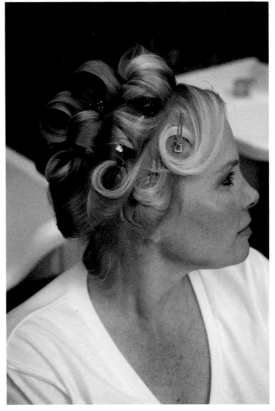

Make it last!

or duckbill clip before you move on to the next section. After you've set (curled and pinned) your hair, allow it to cool before letting it loose. Add a little hair spray to your set for even more holding power.

Two Important Things to Know About Curling Your Hair

1. Curling hair toward the face looks great if you're re-creating the vintage Hollywood look that Veronica Lake and Jean Harlow made famous. Tight curls toward the face also work on tighter naturally curly hair, following the natural curl pattern, like Charlene's in this photo. Otherwise, curling your hair toward your face can leave you looking like the Mandrell sisters did in the *eighties*. That looked great—then.

2. If you're after the current, effortless, tangible "bombshell" wave you've seen on Jessica Simpson, Eva Longoria, and many others, including the Victoria's Secret models, then the hair is curled back and away from the face in barrel curls or loose waves. I use two ways to achieve this look that can also be combined and varied: You can either

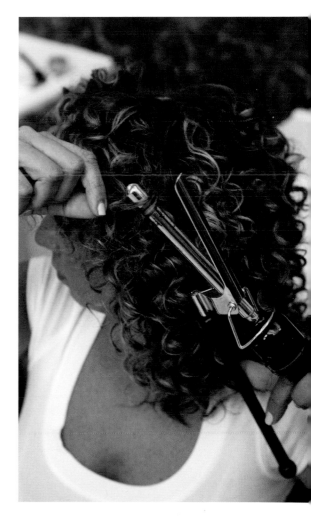

Curling hair toward the face works beautifully on Charlene's naturally curly hair.

curl the hair up and back, away from the face, or curl it down and back from the face. I like to combine both. Everything below the occipital bone (in the middle of the back of the head) is curled up and back, away from the face, and everything above the occipital bone is curled down and back. Va-va-voom!

Boho Chic Curls

I also love very natural-looking, organic curls that are less *pin-up* and more *Boho* (bohemian) *chic*. These curls look more lived-in and less "done." The way to achieve this look is with less volume and by not following the curl all the way to the ends. As always, you should begin on dry hair and prep the hair with a thermal setting spray. Then take random sections, pointing the end of the iron down, and wrap hair around the barrel of the iron. Begin wrapping at the midshaft, which will give you that lived-in, less voluminous look. Wrap the hair down and back, without closing the clamp. Closing the clamp flattens the curl, giving it a very "done" feeling. Leaving the clamp open allows the curls to be more random and less uniform. Leave an inch and a half to two inches of the ends of the hair off

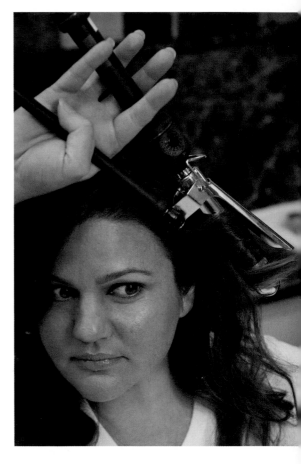

Keeping the ends off the iron gives a relaxed, lived-in look.

the barrel. This gives the ends a straighter look, as if the curl has fallen out, adding to the "undone" vibe. Slide the iron barrel down and further into the hair right before you release it from the barrel. This stretches out the curl, giving the illusion of a lived-in curl.

You can also accomplish a similar curl with your flat iron. Start the same way as above and then point the flat iron up or down and wrap your hair back around one arm of the flat iron. Close the iron without using too much pressure and slide it down the length of the wrapped hair, opening the arms of the iron just before you get to the end. This leaves the ends unfinished for a very loose and natural look.

Beach Waves

One of the looks for which I'm known is beach hair. (I also like to call it bedroom or sex kitten hair.) It's casually curled and tousled and just messy enough! The Boho chic curl has a similar vibe to beach waves. It's all about the texture. Beach hair (even straight hair) looks like it spent a day near saltwater whipping around in the wind. You can create this look easily. Once you have set or styled your hair, flip your head over and lightly spray a volumizer or beach spray into your roots. Either rough up your roots with your hands only, or add a little warm heat with a dryer. The moisture from the volumizer or beach spray on dry hair will cause the cuticle of the hair to swell, much like it would at the beach. Roughing up your roots adds even more texture. You still want to look put together—not like you were in a wind tunnel—so avoid roughing up the ends of your hair. You can always finish with shine serum on your ends and, optionally, a light spray for hold. Flip your head over and use your fingers to style your hair. If you want less volume but the same beach texture, do the same thing without flipping your head over; just tilt it to each side and spray into your roots and rough them up.

Loose Waves

A really great trick to getting a beautiful loose wave can easily be adapted to any of these styles. Before wrapping your hair back and around the iron, try gently twisting the section of hair forward (only the middle part of the length, not the root or end). No matter what size barrel you are using, this will create a looser, more relaxed curl pattern— more of a true wave.

What *real women* have to say about...

Their Curls

"I don't do the salon thing," says Charlene. *"Once in a while I get my hair blow-dried straight. But mostly I wear it curly. But it's a two-hour process to get the look I like and have the curls defined. I wash it, put leave-in products on my hair, and let it air-dry. Air-drying takes a long time."*

Sarah M. *says, "Before I knew Ken, I used to tell everyone that I wanted Ken Paves hair and I copied the hair he did for Carmen Electra and Jessica Simpson. I loved the way their hair looked. I would either curl it back, all in the same direction, or curl it back in one direction and then in the other direction, which gives you a little more volume. If you curl it back in one direction, you brush it out and it gives you this smooth, natural wave. It looks great."*

Bouncy Curls

If you're looking for classic, bouncy curls, try a traditional barrel curl set. Begin at your crown, using a curling iron with an inch or inch and a half barrel. The sections at your crown should be two and a half to three inches wide by an inch to an inch and a half deep. Spray each section with a thermal setting spray and curl back and pin in place (as described above). Work your way back and down to your nape. Continue on the side of your head. There will usually be two rows on each side, one above your ear and one behind. Curl all the sections on each side of your head down, pinning each in place. This look can also be achieved with hot rollers or even Velcro rollers. It creates a contemporary take on the überglamorous big hair that is often associated with the 1960s and 1980s.

A Curling Short Cut

When you're in a hurry, curl only the hair that you see (don't worry about the bottom layers of your hair that are out of view). If your hair is naturally wavy or curly, grab and curl random ends or areas where the curl needs refining. If your hair is straight, curl only from the midshaft to the ends of your underneath hair. Focus on the hair that's easiest for you to reach and curl—the crown and sides.

Enhancing Curly Hair

Curly hair is the most forgiving, since it already has texture, so you can use the curling iron in the most random way and your hair will still end up looking beautiful and natural. Naturally curly hair *can* be curled forward if that's your natural curl pattern.

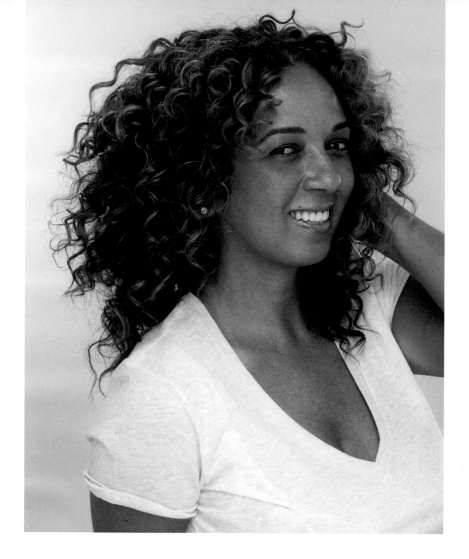

Wrapping your hair around a small barrel without clamping it down will give you a natural look. Wrapping hair around the barrel and clamping it down gives you a more set-looking curl.

When enhancing curly hair, as I did for Charlene during our shoot, I curled the hair forward. I randomly curled her ends and her crown sections, adding volume, more texture, and dimension. I finished her hair by adding shine serum to her curls. The job took about ten minutes. This is something she often does for herself after she air-dries her naturally curly hair or on days in between washings.

CURLING IRONS AND FLAT IRONS

I cannot say this often enough: Healthy hair is the key to any great look. When you are using a curling iron or flat iron, you need to realize that heat-styling damaged hair will only damage it more. This is why you should not blow-dry your hair every day. The same recommendation applies to ironing. Curling and flat ironing are best done infrequently and on healthy hair.

Flat Ironing 101

Here are five really important things to remember when using a flat iron:

1. Make sure your hair is 100 percent dry before you touch your hair with the flat iron. Otherwise you will BURN it.

2. Always use a thermal protective spray, which acts as a barrier between your hair and the heat from the flat iron. The spray also helps lock in your style. After you spray it on, give it a second to dry before using the flat iron. Make sure the spray has dried before ironing!

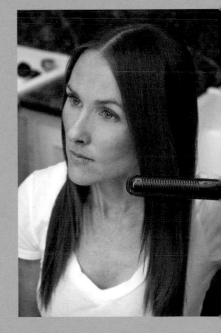

3. Keep the flat iron moving constantly. Don't hold the iron on your hair—slide it down the hair shaft—or you will burn your hair. Clamping and holding your hair in the flat iron will cause long-term breakage and damage. People tend to use a lot more pressure when flat ironing than curling. Keep it moving. Go section by section. For smoother results, make sure to comb or brush each section before you flat iron it.

If you have straight hair, you can normally focus the flat iron on hair from your midshaft down. If you have curly or wavy hair, start at the root and slide the iron down to your ends.

4. Choose the right temperature. Fine hair needs less heat, medium hair requires slightly more heat, and coarse hair requires the most heat. I recommend working with less heat along with steady and controlled movement. The coarser or thicker your hair, the thinner the sections you will want to take.

5. Do not touch your hair until it has cooled. To lock in the straightening, allow each section of your hair to fully cool down.

The Ever-Elegant Chignon

A chignon is essentially a bun—a classic look that takes just a few minutes to achieve. You can wear a chignon at the nape of your neck for a sophisticated look or turn it into an updo for a more glamorous look.

To create a chignon, take an elastic or a hooked rubber band (which I prefer—you can find them in most beauty supply stores and many drugstores) and wrap it around the hair, securing it into a ponytail (see photos). Then simply wrap the length of the ponytail around the base, looser or tighter depending on the look you want. It's that simple. Once you have a shape you like, secure it in place with bobby pins, hairpins, or small butterfly clips. Butterfly clips that are the same color as your hair can sometimes be easier to use than pins. Worn high, medium, or low, this look is great for work, a night out, or a special event.

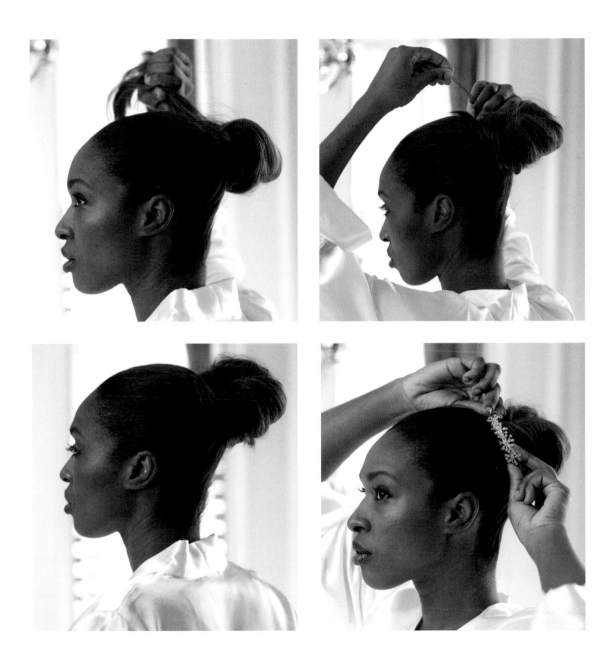

You can accessorize your look with an ornate hair clip.

My Mom's Famous One-Pin French Twist

A French twist is a simple, elegant, and glamorous look that only takes a few minutes to create. I love this look not only for straight hair but also for wavy and curly hair. When my mom's hair is about shoulder-length, she starts doing her French twist. Here's her quick and easy how-to: Gather your hair back as if you were going to put it into a low pony-tail. Twist the hair upward and against the head until you reach the end of the length of your hair. Fold the end of your hair that is not twisted down against your head and tuck it into the twist. Hold this in place. Take a large bobby pin or hairpin and put it through the twist horizontally in the same direction you twisted the hair. Lift the pin off your head while pushing it in against your scalp, flip the pin in the opposite direction, anchoring the hair in place, and slide the pin all the way into the twist. Ooh-la-la, don't you look mighty French!

I love this classic, feminine look. Try it with or without an accessory or headband.

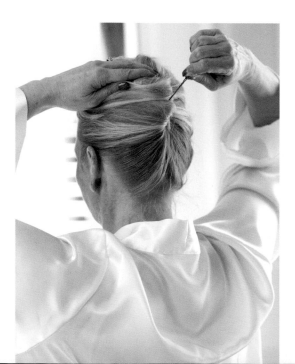
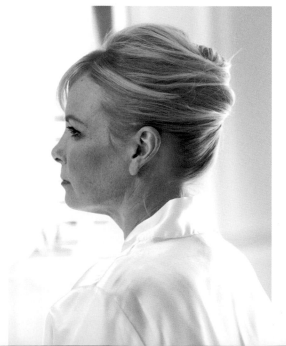

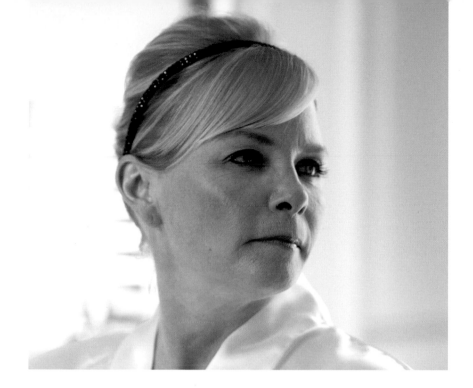

Barrettes, Pins, and Decorative Hair Clips

There are so many things you can do with hair accessories! You can use barrettes, hairpins, and clips to simply keep your hair back and off your face (which is great if you're growing your bangs out) or to dress up a style that you're wearing down and loose.

Hair accessories can take a style from ordinary to formal or flirty, or take a simple look and make it dramatic. Be careful, though; there is a fine line between fashion and foolish. With hair accessories, stay true to you—don't use anything that tries too hard or looks like you borrowed it—and yes, less is usually more. If you're using hair accessories, you may want to choose simple earrings and lose the necklace or bracelet you were thinking of wearing. You don't want to look like you're wearing everything you own all at once.

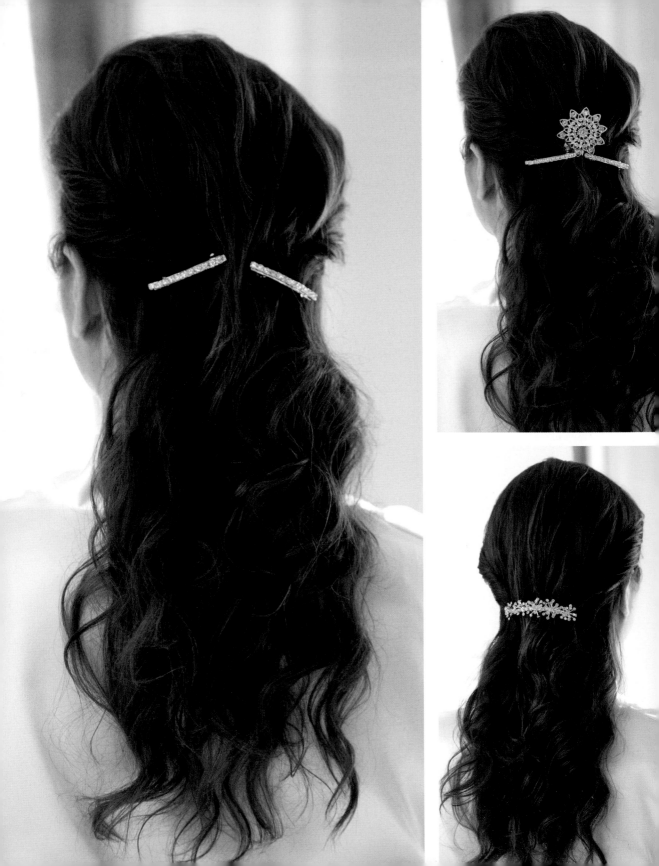

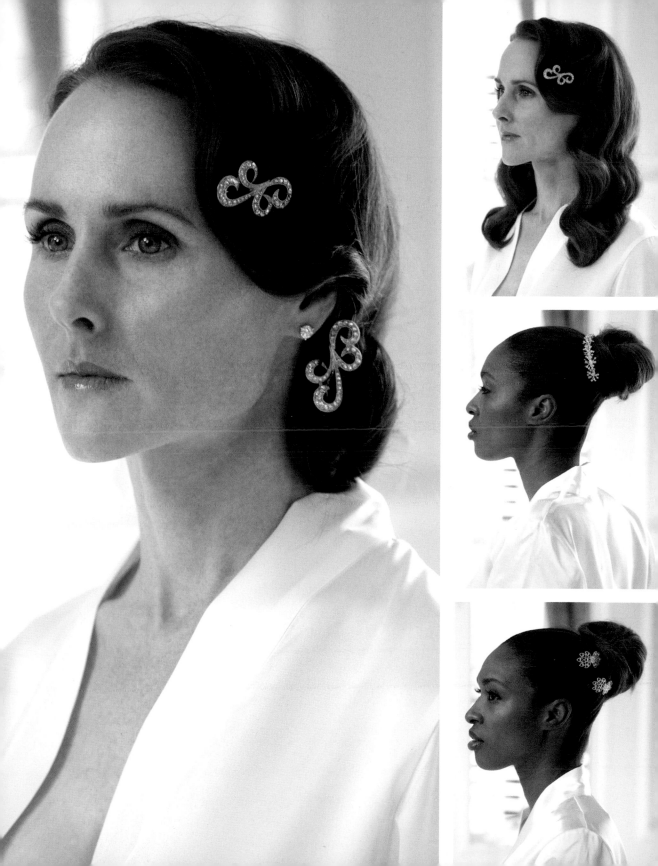

13

Here Comes the Bride

Your wedding day is the greatest, real-life, red-carpet moment you will ever have. If you've been dreaming about this day for a long time, it should be everything you've ever wanted…and more. I always say to a bride, close your eyes and tell me what you look like when you dream about this day. Let's start here. Let's make your dream a reality.

Preparing for the Best Hair Day of Your Life

As a bride-to-be, you have a lot of decisions to make. You have to choose the date and your bridesmaids. You have to find the perfect flowers, invitations, venue, shoes, and, of course, your dream wedding dress. Since it may take some trial and error to get the look you want for your hair on the big day, it's best to get started as quickly as possible, ideally around the same time you've chosen a style for your dress.

Here are some other helpful tips for getting the hair you want on the big day:

- As you're searching for wedding dresses, start to consider hairstyles that look good with the dress. You can never have too many ideas. Preparing ahead of time will help you stay as stress-free as possible. You have enough to do. So have fun with this! Collect images of hairstyles you like from magazines. Rather than trying to remember what you like, it's helpful to show your hairstylist pictures that clearly communicate what you want.

- Not every hairdresser likes to do formal styles. If your regular stylist feels comfortable styling wedding hair, that's great. If not, ask your stylist to recommend someone. Find a stylist who enjoys doing formal styles but also works well with your hair type.

- Set up an appointment (or a few) for a trial hairstyle. Come equipped with images of what you like—whether it's a style or an accessory. It's more important for the hairstyle to fit you than to fit the dress. Try different ideas that you and your stylist may have and take lots of pictures. Also remind your stylist that whatever look you choose has to last!

- Time your last haircut and/or color before your big day. You want to give your hair enough time (usually a week or two in advance) to settle but still look fresh.

- Although I always advocate that you do whatever will make you feel beautiful, I suggest that on this day you also take into consideration how the love of your life, who will be waiting for you at the end of the aisle, loves to see you look. There is nothing to compare with the first moment you see each other on that memorable day.

- Consider the location of your wedding and the climate. A beach wedding may not be the best place for a sculpted updo or the best time to smooth your curls.

- Remember you will be looking at your wedding pictures for years to come. How many of your friends have looked at their wedding pictures and said, "Oh my God, look at my hair! Well, those were the the eighties (or whenever)!" Whether romantic, classic, Old Hollywood glam, or sleek and modern, keep your look timeless, not trendy.

- Don't try something so drastic that it leaves everyone wondering who that is walking down the aisle.

- Choose a look that makes you feel like the princess you always dreamed of being. Confidence is the best accessory you can wear on your wedding day.

Choosing Your Wedding Hairstyle

It is so important that you feel beautiful and comfortable today. There are many things to take into consideration when deciding how you will wear your hair on your wedding day! The first thing to consider is what makes you feel the best. If you never wear your hair up because you don't like the way it looks, then maybe an updo just isn't for you, and that's OK. If you always wear your hair very straight, maybe today is not the day to try tight curls. I have heard from many disappointed brides who, on the day of their wedding (having skipped a hair trial), got a combination of both. I call this the "pineapple"—the look that you see all too often on brides, where the hair is put into small curls, pulled very high and tight, the curls plopped on top of your head and shellacked into place. You know the look—it's like your mom's prom hair and looks like it requires a floral spray of baby's breath. I am here to tell you that you have other options. Wedding hair today is far more personal and tailored just for you, to make you look and feel great—it's all about the individual! Many of the hairstyles I've shown you, in Chapter 12 for example, are tailored to a wide variety of hair types and would also work as beautiful bride or bridesmaids' hair.

The Hair Makes the Dress

Three brides may wear the same dress and yet look totally different—it's the hair that really sets them apart. When we used to think of wedding hair, the elegant updo usually came to mind. I am still a huge fan and believe that no one rocks an updo like Jennifer Lopez, a look I have created on her many times. An updo, whether it's high or low, sculpted or casual and loose, is a signature formal look that works well with all dress styles and necklines, especially a high neckline.

More and more we are seeing brides wearing their hair down, soft and natural. There is something so chic about seeing a woman who looks effortlessly like herself on her wedding day. Soft, casual hair is beautiful with a simple dress, but it can also be just the right touch when everything else is formal. If you wear your hair down, however, it should look very healthy and luxurious. You can give this style some flair, and even make it work with a high neckline, by pinning one or both sides of your hair back. A simple brooch or an ornate hair accessory can add even more glamour. Hair that is half up can be very romantic, too.

If you love Old Hollywood glamour, put some in your style! This look is timeless and classic. A soft retro wave is great, whether you're wearing your hair up or down. You can go all the way or add just a subtle hint of a wave. The faux retro bob can really glamorize your style.

A cascading ponytail is another good option if you don't want to wear all of your hair up, but still want to have some movement.

Where you part your hair can also define your style. Try a center-parted low ponytail, or a deep side part with Veronica Lake waves or a side chignon. Maybe you like your hair parted down the middle, worn down and cascading behind your shoulders.

The texture of your hair also influences your style. Curls tend to evoke a romantic feeling while straight hair is sleeker. Choose what

Bridesmaid Hair

Weddings are similar to fashion shows. There are lots of girls and only one bride at the end of the show. One thing that helps fashion shows look so spectacular is that there is a common theme to all the models' hair. Whether you and your bridesmaids choose a similar texture or possibly a similar style, this common element will help keep the look of your wedding chic and elegant.

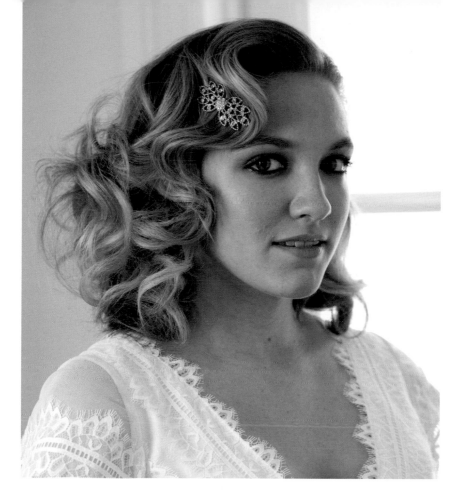

Caitlin's romantic curls perfectly complement the vintage look of her dress,

feels and looks most beautiful to you. Maybe you want a wavy half-up Bardot style or a beautiful wavy texture that's pulled back, à la Grace Kelly. Or maybe a sleek French twist or a straight-flowing sheet of hair is your style.

Wherever you find your inspiration, whatever makes you feel beautiful, I encourage you to walk down the aisle as your best you. There is nothing more breathtaking than a bride coming down the aisle glowing, radiant, confident, and comfortable in her own skin—a vision of her own loveliness.

What *real women* have to say about...

Being Brides for a Day

We had so much fun turning Caitlin and Nyke into brides for the day. Caitlin's dress was simple with a vintage flair. We decided to go for a modern take on an Old Hollywood look. *"I love this look,"* said Caitlin. *"It's so beautiful."*

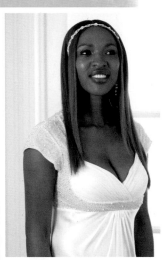

When Lisa saw her daughter in a wedding dress, with her hair and makeup done, she took a step back and said, *"You are so beautiful."*

Even I had to take a step back when I saw Caitlin dressed as a bride. She looked stunning, like a princess, but I realized she wasn't my "little" princess anymore. She looked like a beautiful young woman who will one day make a very lovely bride.

Nyke's dress was also vintage inspired, but with a sleeker, simpler style. I like the irony of the sleek hair with the vintage dress. We tied it together by adding a vintage-inspired headband into Nyke's sleek hairstyle. The end result was a very feminine, Boho chic vibe.

"I also loved the bridal dress," says Nyke. *"It was one of my favorite looks that day! White always makes me look very native, which is nice. I loved the headband. It reminded me of the olden days. Maybe Cleopatra."*

Mad for Makeup

Just as a good hair day gives you a lift, makeup can make you feel better instantly. A little concealer, mascara, or a pop of color on your lips can brighten your look—and attitude—in seconds. The fresh face you see in the mirror and present to the world helps you embrace the beautiful woman you are.

Accepting and Enhancing Your Unique Beauty

Like hair, makeup is meant to enhance the features you love and camouflage areas that need a little extra TLC. But it's not about hiding behind your makeup. So many women layer on the makeup to hide from the world. They may go for layer upon layer of foundation or tons of heavy eye makeup. Piling on makeup can date your look and even age you.

There's a time and place to amp things up, makeup-wise. But not for an everyday look.

Beauty, to me, should never be about hiding. Simple makeup is current, modern, and fresh. It's all about accepting and enhancing your unique beauty and being the best you that you can be.

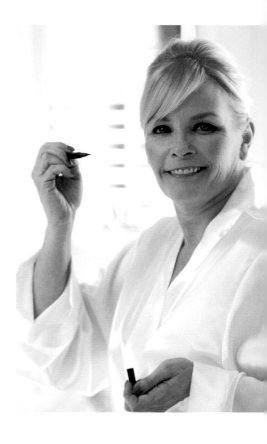

The Best Foundation for Makeup

Makeup looks best on glowing, luminous skin. The keys to always looking beautiful are healthy skin and shiny hair. I tell all my clients to follow a good skin regimen of cleansing and moisturizing.

A healthy diet of fresh fruits and vegetables, as well as olive oil, salmon, nuts, and seeds (which are full of omega-3 fatty acids, which make your skin and hair glow), is critical. So is drinking lots of water to hydrate your hair and skin. Moving your body and sweating out those toxins is one of the best things you can do to keep your skin supple and young-looking. Vitamins and supplements that help your hair and skin stay healthy and your nails grow thicker are good for the rest of your body, too.

Once you've looked in the mirror and embraced your freshly cleansed and moisturized skin, you can start thinking about makeup. It's key to love what you see before you even get started, because what you see in the mirror is you.

What *real women* have to say about . . .

Makeup

"I'll get dressed up for a major event, but normally I don't wear any makeup except a little lipstick—a dull rose," says Afton. *"I wear the same one every time. I put my makeup on in the car—the only time I ever put it on. I do like to do my nails with sparkly gels, though, partly because it protects my nails when I work in the garden."*

"I'm sooooo into taking care of every inch of my body," says Charlene. *"Anyone who knows me knows my bathroom looks like a Neiman Marcus counter. My beauty regimen is to eat healthy, drinks lots of water—and coconut water. I love a great moisturizer . . . I'm not big on tons of makeup—I love sun-kissed skin with dewy cheeks and tousled hair, fresh off the runway. I love bronzer mascaras. And lip-gloss and eyelash curlers are a must!"*

Beauty on the Run— Around Town and at Work

OK. You put your hair up into a cute ponytail and only have five minutes—if that—for makeup. Your makeup routine doesn't have to be complicated. No matter how much time you have—or don't have—you can still feel better with just a little bit of makeup. When you have more time, you can relax and enjoy the process more.

One of the looks I love, and which you can achieve in five minutes flat, is fresh, dewy skin with softly colored lips and a little mascara, paired, of course, with beautiful hair.

One of my favorite tricks, which I learned a long time ago, is to mix your foundation with a light, facial moisturizer. This gives you a sheer, clean base. You can then build on this with concealer to take care of any problem spots, such as dark, under-eye circles or the area just below your nose, which can tend to show redness. Add a little powder for oil control.

Mascara is another must for an on-the-go look. A little bit goes a long way. Swish a little on your lashes to make your eyes pop and give them more definition. Honestly, that's all you need for everyday errand-running makeup. If you need an extra boost, add a soft eyeliner and bronzer or blush for some extra color. As for work, the key is to look polished and professional.

WHENEVER MY MOM IS GOING ON TV or before the camera, I know she feels so much better with flawless-looking skin. If we're in a rush, I'll grab her moisturizer, squirt a little in my hand, add some of her foundation, and apply it to her skin. It evens out her complexion and gives her skin a sheer natural look, which she loves. I've done this too, when I've gone on camera, just minutes before getting to the set. I've applied this mixture while I was walking. My skin looked great. This is something you can do in two seconds.

Lip-Gloss and Lipstick

Lip-gloss is a life-saver that can pull your whole look together and make you look polished. And it's always sexy. A high gloss can be too much for everyday wear so I suggest saving it for nighttime. A regular gloss gives you just enough shimmer. Remember—everyday makeup is all about subtly enhancing your natural beauty.

For work or for an everyday look, I like tawny pinks for lips, which work with all complexions. This is a basic shade every woman should have in her handbag. An earthy pink adds just enough color to give your lips a healthy glow.

Lipstick to me means business. It usually gives your lips a heavy look. For everyday beauty, think fresh and natural—save the lipstick for nighttime.

Bronzers, Highlighters, and Blush

Look for bronzers and highlighters in similar tones. Using lighter and darker shades of your base color will allow you to create a natural-looking, tone-on-tone contour. For example, you can highlight and draw attention to a particular facial feature—your cheekbones, for example— by making them look more prominent. To accomplish this, use a color that's a shade or two lighter than your base color.

A darker shade, on the other hand, helps to shadow, minimize, and contour areas you don't love. If you put a darker shade under your chin, for instance, it will contour your jawline, making your face, neck, and chin look slimmer instantly.

Blush makes your skin look fresh and radiant. Pick a shade with pink hues to give you a rosy glow. It will make you look healthy and younger, too!

Oh, You Sexy Mama!

Now it's time to have some fun! I love glamorous makeup for the right occasion. Two of my favorite movies that give me "event" hair and makeup inspiration are *Mahogany*, with Diana Ross, and *The Eyes of Laura Mars*, with Faye Dunaway. Both women are striking in these iconic films that represent times when women really embraced and celebrated their femininity. The women portrayed were strong and confidant—and boy, were they glamorous!

One of the best tips I've learned from helping get women ready for the red carpet is knowing when to play up makeup and when to hold back. If you're focusing on and playing up one area, then go light everywhere else. This helps to keep your look balanced and less theatrical, unless you're hitting the stage, in which case, give it all you got!

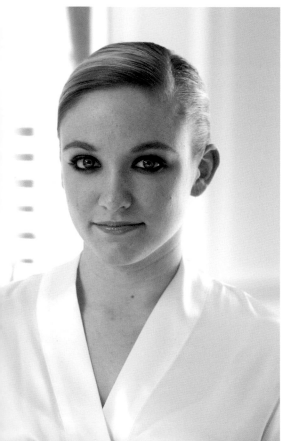

- If makeup is your focus, your hair should be simple and take backstage (did I really just say that?).

- If you go heavy or dramatic with your eyes, go with a nude, pale pink, or natural lip. Dramatic eyes and lips together are too overpowering.

- If you go for a bold lip color, go with a soft, more natural eye. A cream-colored shadow with mascara and a little liner on your lid could be all you need, or just a simple sixties line above your eye.

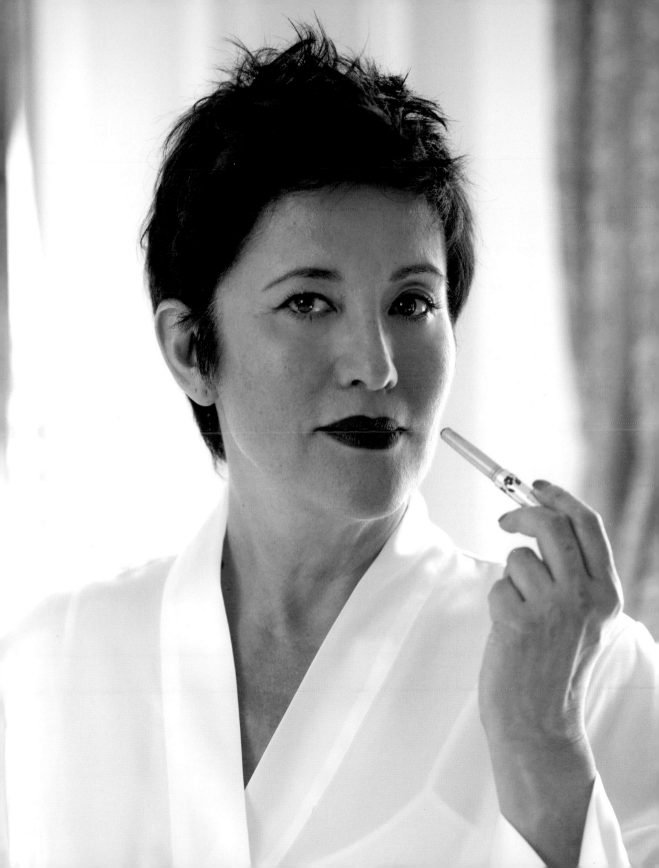

SARAH LUCERO ON MAKEUP

If anyone knows makeup, it's my good friend, celebrity makeup artist Sarah Lucero, who is the Stila Cosmetics (gorgeous!) spokesperson and Global Director of Creative Artistry. She has done makeup for everyone from Brooke Shields to Victoria and David Beckham. Sarah, who is one of the nicest people I know, makes everyone she works with look absolutely beautiful.

Here are Sarah's beauty basics:

Take good care of your skin. Beautiful makeup starts with beautiful skin. Cleansing, moisturizing, and using products like Retinol are critical for good skin.

As a makeup artist I feel you need to exfoliate often and moisturize daily. Scrubs are a must. Invest in a Clarisonic skin care brush system to wash your face daily. It truly changes the way you cleanse your skin.

The right tools are important. Good-quality brushes allow you to properly blend and control the application of your makeup. Everyone should invest in a good foundation brush, a double-sided eye-shadow brush, and a smoky liner brush. I have three brushes in my personal makeup bag and could easily do my clients' makeup with these three tools. You also need a good-quality eyelash curler for lashes. This is a must! Other than that, fingers make the best beauty tools.

Tips for looking your best when you are on the run. The best products to have on hand for the days you are on the run are products that multi-task. Double-duty beauty products that do more than one thing will save you time. I suggest tinted moisturizer or illuminating powder foundation with SPF added in the formula. You can save time and skip a couple of steps with either complexion product.

I also suggest a cream blush compact that can be applied to lips and cheeks for a "flush of youth" and a touch of natural color. I also love to use lip and cheek stains when I'm on the run. They last longer and tend to stay put so you don't have to look in the mirror so often. Plus they are easy to apply with your fingertips.

A nice "day" look when you have a little more time. Invest in a natural eye shadow palette that allows you to create a modern and balanced makeup look. Many brands have palettes available that combine natural, bronze, shimmer, and matte shadows so you can enhance and correct your eyes and bring attention to them in a modern way.

I also like the idea of using a concealer to brighten and correct the under-eye area and balance out any redness in the skin. Look for a creamy liquid concealer. The best textures are available in a click pen. These types of formulas are usually sheer and blend in effortlessly.

Beautiful makeup always starts with beautiful skin. If you have a few extra minutes to get ready, you should focus on polishing up your complexion and adding a cream blush to the apples of your cheeks. Always enhance your brows with a tinted brow gel. You will look feminine, youthful, and totally put together all day long!

Getting ready for work. Depending on what you do for a living, always go for a balanced and harmonious look. Try and look polished by wearing products that enhance and bring out your best features. I suggest a great sheer lip color and lip-gloss, a coral or pink cheek color, and lined eyes in a bronze or gray liner, with a couple of coats of mascara for daily work makeup. That way you look like the best version of yourself. You can always up the glam factor for work events after hours and company parties! You should also ask the makeup artist behind the counter of your favorite brand to show you new trends, every season, to update your seasonal beauty wardrobe and look.

When you're preparing for conservative events or meetings, I suggest a powder foundation to smooth out any redness and keep shine away. You want to look put together and polished. If you have on too much bronzer or a shimmer highlight, it could tend to look greasy and distract from your presentation. Wear a makeup look that makes you feel really comfortable and confident.

Getting ready for a night out. This is the time to shine! Wear a shimmery jewel-tone shadow on eyelids to bring out your eyes and catch attention. Layer an extra coat of black mascara and even wear a few false lashes to bring your eyes out.

Branch out and wear a navy or deep plum eye shadow or liner for a smoky-eyed look, rather than the expected black or gray. Try wearing a bold sparkle waterproof liquid liner if you will be out dancing all night—this way your makeup will stay perfectly in place all night long.

Going for all-out glam. Super glam makeup is a bit more serious and dramatic. Play with a wine-stained lip and contoured cheek. I prefer powder cheek-contour shades. They are easy to blend. You can easily control the application of a contour shade with a brush.

Eyes can be strong and heavily lined with pencil or cream liner in a bold shade like black, bronze, or gray. Brows should be polished and groomed, but not too dark. Try a tinted brow gel to lift and brighten your natural brow hair and create a fuller, youthful-looking brow.

I suggest you allow your complexion to remain sheer and a bit glossy and dewy. Use an illuminating tinted moisturizer to brighten your complexion rather than a heavy foundation. This way you can play with different textures on the eyes, skin, lips, and cheeks.

■ The Cat Eye

This trend is huge, so I suggest investing in a high-quality liquid liner in black. Everyone can wear liquid liner. It's all about finding the right product and placing it in just the right spot to suit your eye shape.

Trace a line along top lashes and apply mascara to freshly curled lashes to achieve this look. Leave the rest of your eye bare and clean.

Here's a little secret I always like to share: Try applying your mascara first before you apply the liquid liner. This way you can see exactly where you should start—and end—your liner.

Opt for a fresh cheek color and sheer nude gloss for a finished look.

■ The Doe Eye

I love creating wide doe eyes by concentrating the liner in the center of the lower lash line and sweeping it along the rest of the lashes. Find the widest area of your eyes and drag the line out a bit with a deep matte coco shade.

The key is to restructure the shape of your eyes by enhancing and contouring. Create the shape you want to see rather than always following the shape you have. It's all about balancing and correcting features.

The last step: Load on mascara in the center of the top and bottom lashes. I'm a fan of mascara and when in doubt I always add a little more!

The right makeup to wear with retro Hollywood hair, chignons, sleek ponytails, and other evening styles. Red matte lips are the secret beauty element to tie this look together. Look for velvet textures of classic red lipstick and deepen it by using a lip pencil or lip stain as a base. Keep the rest of your makeup clean. Enhance your dramatic lips by using neutral tones for the rest of your makeup.

Keep the intensity of your eye makeup along the top lash line to bring out the shape of your eyes. You have to focus on your favorite feature and edit the rest. This allows your makeup to remain timeless and very sophisticated.

■ The Smoky Eye

Step 1: Apply a natural shadow as an all-over eye base from lash line to brow bone. This will smooth out the surface texture of your eyelids and camouflage uneven lids. This also allows all other eye shadows to glide on effortlessly and easily.

Step 2: Dip a medium-size brush into the shadow (I prefer espresso, deep brown, or bronze shades). Apply to the entire lid and blend into the crease. Wrap the same shade under the entire lower lash line to create diffusion and a smoky effect. This is called "wrapping" the eye.

Step 3: Apply a medium matte shadow to the crease of your eye to contour and gently define, which brings out the shape of your eyes. Keep your eyes open and look straight into the mirror for a flawless application. This will allow you to place the shadow in the most flattering space right above your natural crease. Blend "up" rather than back and forth.

Step 4: Line your eyes with a creamy kohl pencil on your water line— the inner rim of your eye—and just under the lower lash line. Use a small liner brush to gently sweep off any pigment from the pencil tip and buff that into the lash line for a true diffused, smoky, defined eye. Finish this look with two or three coats of mascara on the top and bottom lashes.

The right lipstick to wear when you're playing up your eyes or lips.

• If you're playing up your lips, with a dark, smoky eye, wear a pink or nude glossy lip color. Keeping the lips soft allows the eyes to stand out and hold more makeup in a modern style.

• If you're playing up your lips, keep your eyes soft and simple. Try a hot pink or coral lipstick or wear a cream blush on your lips for a tinted-stain effect. Always keep the cheek and lip color in the same color family; otherwise your makeup may look outdated.

A soft but dramatic evening look. I love using soft grays on the eyes and creating a fuzzy, diffused, smoky look. Try a pastel pink on cheeks and lips for a sultry vintage effect. Deepen the lash line with shadow rather than heavy liner. It will be dramatic but not dark.

■ How to put on false eyelashes.
Apply mascara first and then layer strip lashes or false individual lashes against your natural lash line. Use Duo Eyelash Adhesive in the dark tone. Let the glue sit for about 60 seconds and then apply the lashes. The glue needs to be tacky to adhere to the eyelid.

Most women need to trim the lash strips to fit their eye shape. You can clip off the end of the band with scissors, if needed. Do this before you apply the glue.

The All-Important Brow

When I've done makeovers on *The Oprah Winfrey Show* and *The Biggest Loser*, I've actually heard women gasp when they've had their brows groomed, shaped, and even dyed! One woman was so pleased with her new look, she said, "Ken! I look like I just had a face-lift!"

Another woman I helped make over wrote to me afterward, saying how much she loved the cut I gave her. People kept telling her, "You look better than I've ever seen you. There's something different about you…" She wrote, "Ken, it was the hair—and the brows. They changed my whole look. I feel like a movie star!"

That's how I want you to feel, too. Well-groomed, well-shaped eyebrows are as important as the right makeup and hair. The right brow can change your whole look by taking you from ordinary to stunning. As with hair and makeup, it's all about tweaking things a bit and changing things up to enhance what you already have. Do you have to shape your brows? No. But I promise you, you will love the end result.

SARAH LUCERO ON BROWS

Brows frame the face and can easily transform your look. Most women can update their look and even appear younger by simply brushing their brows with a tinted brow gel and filling in sparse areas with a brow pen.

Go a shade lighter than your natural brow hair. Focus on shading and creating a shadow of fullness behind your brow hair. If you have thin ends, only add product to that area. You will see your brows balance out and look complete just by adding a small amount of product to the correct spot.

216

Clothes

DO MAKE
THE WOMAN!

The clothes you wear can reveal a lot about how you feel about yourself. I'm not talking about the hot brand you may be wearing at the moment or the fact that you always sport the latest trend—but how you wear your clothes and the shapes you've chosen for yourself.

Women who wear clothes that are too tight or skirts that are up to *there* may think they look hot and sexy, but their clothes may actually be saying something quite different! On the other hand, always wearing clothes that are too loose or too long can suggest that you're hiding something—or that you just don't care.

Just like your hair, your clothes can showcase what you like about your figure and camouflage what you may not. Finding clothes that work with your shape is yet another way to feel better about yourself. Thick, thin, tall, short, curvy, or not—stand proud and show folks what you've got and tell them it's all right!

In order to properly dress your body, though, you have to realize what it really looks like and accept it, just as you have done with your hair.

I want you to love and embrace your body. All of it. If you don't find yourself beautiful, no one else will. While you're certainly not going to show up at your neighbor's Super Bowl party or your sister's wedding *au natural*, like Lady Godiva, it's still important to accept and love what's underneath your clothes. The real you is under those clothes, so you need to love what's there.

Get Naked!

The next time you are finished taking a shower or bath, drop your towel and look in the mirror, just like you did in the beginning of the book. I know, I know. This could be difficult. Don't cover your eyes or just take a glimpse. Take a good look. Check out the back side, too. Do you have a hand mirror? Do a couple of side bends, turn around, reach for something. Hey, stop sucking in your stomach. Get acquainted with what you really look like. This will help you get to know the areas you like the most about your body and want to enhance with the way you dress.

As you stand before yourself, in your birthday suit, take it all in. Look yourself in the eyes and say, "I AM BEAUTIFUL!" Say it until you truly believe it. Shout it out. When you believe that you really are beautiful—skinny arms, rounded tummy, saddlebags, flat bum, whatever it is you see—you will feel confident in your skin.

See? That wasn't so bad. This is you. And you, my love, are beautiful.

Getting dressed will just be the icing on the cake, knowing the true beauty of what's underneath it all.

A friend once told me, when she saw a picture of herself, "If that's what I really look like, then shoot me. That is disgusting." My heart broke for her. She is beautiful. Her reaction to the photo came from years of disregarding herself and being afraid to see the truth. I actually thought she was one of the most confident women I knew. She had no idea what she really looks like and how beautiful she actually is.

I am writing this book for women like my friend, who are terrorized into avoiding reality by the unrealistic pressure to look a certain way that they themselves cannot even accept. I have worked very hard for almost twenty years to earn a voice as a beauty expert, and I have seen it *all*. I promise you that. I am here to tell you, you are beautiful! Keep reading. You'll get it!

It is important to come to terms with what you love about your body right now—not what you loved twenty years ago and not what you loved before you had kids or gained fifteen pounds, but what you have now. The taut, tight tummy or hot butt you had way back when isn't the tummy or butt you have now. Find out what you love now and work with that. Live in the now. Celebrate yourself now. Be in the present. You're not who you were yesterday. You are who you are today. Get to know yourself!

Wait! I Have a Waist??

Just like with your hair and makeup, figuring out what your best features are—and working with them—is the best way to ensure that you'll always dress in the most flattering way for your particular body shape.

What *real women* have to say about...

What They Love About Their Bodies

During the photo shoots for this book, celebrity stylist Kayla McGee and I wanted to dress the ladies in clothes that showed off their best features. I asked some of the women what they love about their bodies.

"I love my legs because they're long and toned," said Tip, *who wore a purple, figure-hugging jersey dress that showed off her shapely calves. "I like to wear short-length skirts that go to mid-thigh. I wear dresses and skirts most of the time. I rarely wear jeans. I feel constricted in them. But I do like leggings, because they also show off my legs."*

"I love my shoulders because they're strong," said Chloe, who donned a sexy black top that showed off her toned shoulders and beautiful neckline. *"I used to carry a lot on my shoulders. That was my own doing. Now I've learned how to live and let live. My shoulders are now burden-free."*

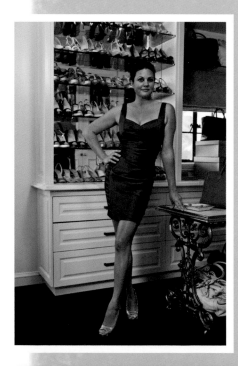
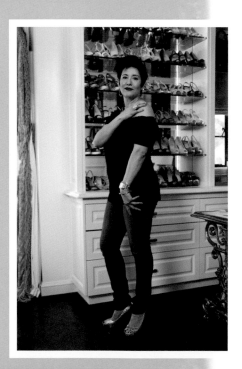

When I asked my sister-in-law, Lisa, what she liked best about her body, she said, *"I don't know."*

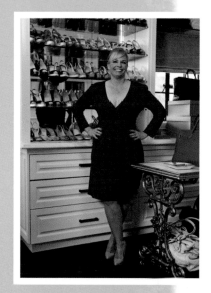

This is a woman I've known for more than thirty years. Lisa started dating my brother when they were in high school. She even babysat for me. (I was a handful, to say the least.) She is an amazing wife and mother who has raised beautiful kids, but like so many other women out there, Lisa couldn't readily say what she loved best about her body.

I knew immediately what her best feature is. I said to her, "Isn't it your waist?" Lisa put her hands on her waist, paused for a moment, and said, "Yes! You're right!" It took me asking her about this for Lisa to realize that she has a sexy waist, which highlights the feminine, hourglass figure my brother loves so much.

Lisa put on a red, figure-hugging dress that Kayla had selected for her. She looked stunning. When she looked in the mirror, she loved what she saw. *"I would never have picked that dress if I were shopping,"* she said. *"I would think it was too dowdy. But when I put it on, it accentuated my curves. What I realize from this is that I love my curves. When I get home, I'm getting a dress like this one to show off my waist."*

When Lisa first saw the color of the dress, she wasn't sure about that, either. *"I've never bought anything that was red,"* she said. *"I didn't think I could wear red as a blonde."* Oh yes, she could. "Striking hues like deep reds and blues look beautiful on blondes," said Kayla.

Seeing these women, who all mean so much to me, realize just how beautiful their bodies are was a pivotal moment for me. This is exactly what I wanted them to see at the photo shoot that day. And it's what I want for you, too.

I want you to ask yourself, "What do I love most about my body? Is it my legs? My arms? My waist? My décolleté?" Whatever it is, that's what I would like you to show the world.

Finding ways to enhance your figure by the way you dress is easy. Look at any woman whose body image you admire and take note of her wardrobe choices. I promise you will recognize a pattern, seeing her play up what she loves best about her figure. If she loves her legs, I am sure she's no stranger to dresses, skirts, shorts, and even skinny jeans and leggings. If she has an überfeminine hourglass figure, I am sure she loves wearing belts and tucks in her tops to accentuate her waist. If a woman doesn't like her waist so much, you may see her go for tops that are longer and looser in the waist, which elongate her torso.

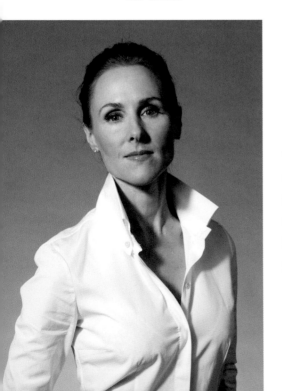

What Every Woman Should Have in Her Closet

Your wardrobe should consist of some basic, classic, and timeless pieces in equally basic, simple, and classic colors. Classic pieces never go out of style. You can easily keep these looks current by building on them, as you transition from season to season and trend to trend, with accessories or one or two pieces that are in fashion right now.

What's great about having timeless pieces in your wardrobe is that you know you have the perfect go-to look for every occasion. By taking time to find clothes that fit your body well and flatter you, you will save yourself time and angst when you get invited to a last-minute cocktail party or dinner. No one likes rushing through a store to find the right dress or pants when you have limited time. That's usually when you end up with something that you'll wear once and then let sit in your closet until the next tag sale.

If you find a dress or pair of pants that you love, but which doesn't fit exactly right, bring it to a tailor for inexpensive, custom fitting to ensure that it will fit you perfectly—whenever you need it.

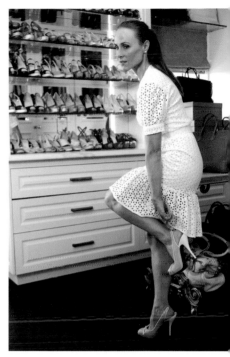

Here is my list of must-haves for every woman:

- A perfect, simple, little black dress that fits beautifully and always makes you look fantastic.

- A simple cream-colored or gray dress. What's great about neutral colors like cream, taupe, grey, brown, and black is that you can accessorize them with the color of the moment, whether it's something bright for spring or a color that's a little richer for fall. You can also dress up these looks with simple, elegant jewelry, a chignon, and a

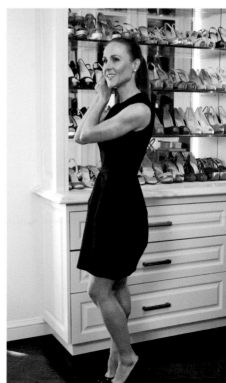

stunning pump, or go more casual with fun jewelry, scarves, hair worn natural and loose, and high-heeled sandals.

◆ Jeans. Today jeans can go everywhere. You can easily dress them up with a sexy top, drop earrings, and heels, or dress them down with a classic T-shirt and flip-flops.

◆ Well-fitting slacks or trousers in neutral colors.

◆ Skirts, long or short—whatever suits your figure and personality best.

◆ A well-fitting black blazer that can go over a beautiful dress or top and give you instant polish. I love blazers in cream, too.

◆ A classic white button-down shirt, which can add elegance to any look. I also love a button-down in black, for a sexier look.

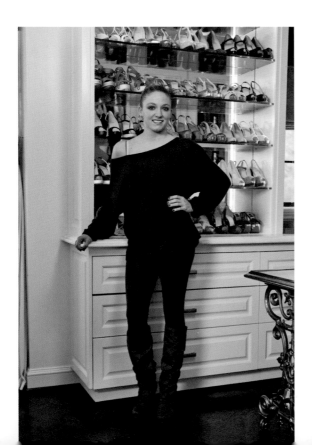
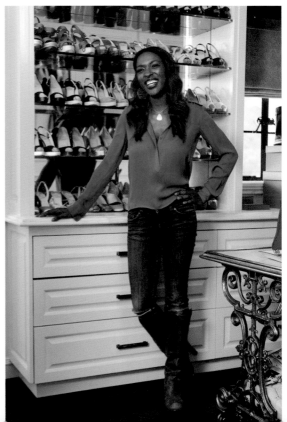

KAYLA McGEE ON CLOTHES

As a celebrity stylist in L.A., Kayla McGee has worked for shows such as *How Do I Look?* and *The X Factor,* where she dressed Paula Abdul. She outfitted the women at the photo shoots for this book, making them look fabulous while maintaining each woman's personal sense of style.

Overall Tips for Dressing the Right Way

- The two things every woman should do when getting dressed are creating an hourglass figure and elongating themselves. Dark wash jeans, for example, always give the illusion of making your legs look long.

- Make sure your clothes fit right.

- Wear Spanx. Everyone does…did I say "everyone"? Because all celebrities do. Those pictures you see on the red carpet? Even the smallest size-0 actress has Spanx (or slimmers) on. They keep everything in place and smooth out your curves.

- Find an actress you like whose body type is similar to yours. Check out what she's wearing on the red carpet and when she's out and about. Most likely she has a stylist, and you can steal her style without the cost of a stylist!

- If you're not happy with your legs, put on a little self-tanner.

- Don't let age stop you from wearing anything—except fluorescent colors and clothes that are too itty-bitty. Those don't really look good on anyone.

- For curvy women: You want to find a jean that hits at the widest part of your leg and then goes straight down. Trouser pants are great for this. Avoid jeans that go in at the knee.

This will only draw the eye to your hips and make them look bigger. Stay away from bell-bottoms and skinny jeans.

- For women who lack curves: Skinny jeans are great for you. We all have curves and this look helps to accentuate the ones you have. A jean that goes in at the knee and then out into a bell or boot-cut shape is also a great cut for you because it's adding curves and creating that hourglass shape you want.

- If you have a busty chest: Stay away from boat-neck shirts or anything that adds more volume up top. You want to elongate your neck. V-neck or scoop neck shirts are great for you. Throwing on a jacket with a built-in waist highlights the smallest part of your figure—your waist—and helps create that hourglass look. (I always love a white tank under button-up shirts or cardigans because the white draws the eye up to the face and brightens it.)

- For women with flatter chests: Voluminous shirts and blouses are perfect for you. So are shirts with ruffles at the top, which help to create that hourglass look for you.

The Perfect Little Black Dress for Every Body Shape.

- If you're curvy: A wrap dress is perfect for you. You want to pick a dress that wraps around your waist to accentuate it. Wrap dresses create a nice V-neck, which elongates the neck and body.

- If you lack curves: You want a dress with a high neckline that cinches at the waist with a voluminous, full skirt. It's very Audrey Hepburn and gives you an hourglass shape—like the little black dress Sarah M. wore at our shoot (see page 223).

- If you're tall: A long column dress is a pretty option for you.

Body Image

If you're not at your "ideal" weight (and let's be honest—who really is?), please do not use this as an excuse not to look fabulous! First off, if you look good, you feel good…if you feel good, you're more likely to reach your goals…like losing weight. Wherever you are in life, you deserve to look your best. The key to looking good, no matter what size you are, is wearing clothes that fit just right. I've seen size-4 women who have muffin tops because their jeans are too tight and cut too low. I've also seen women who look like they've lost twenty pounds simply by wearing a structured jacket—as opposed to the loose tops they were wearing to cover up their weight.

Adding more fabric and volume doesn't cover up any extra weight you might be carrying. Instead, it makes you look bigger. If you're not happy with your tummy and you're wearing a shirt with a lot of extra fabric and then covering that with an ill-fitting sweater, you're adding the illusion of an extra ten pounds to the area you think you're hiding.

Instead, throw on a more slimming, fitted, dark or bright colored cardigan with a white tank top underneath. The eye will be drawn to the bright color of your sweater and the pop of white from the tank—not to your tummy. (Bright colors are happy colors. Try wearing an orange top instead of the drab black or gray you're used to wearing and then tell me how your day goes. I promise you will feel a lot brighter and happier.)

Besides well-fitting cardigans, you can also go for a structured jacket that nips at the waist, highlighting your waist and curves. Trust me. Try it and see how you feel.

An Instant Feel-Good Tip

If you're truly not happy with the way you're feeling and looking because you haven't lost that extra weight yet, put on your favorite outfit, spend an extra five minutes on your hair, take the time to put on mascara and lipstick, and I guarantee you'll feel better and have a more positive outlook on your day and your body.

Tips for Dressing Well at Every Age

* In Your Twenties. Your twenties are all about discovering who you are and figuring out your personal style. For the first time in your life, you're on your own. You're no longer under your parents' wing. You're working now and starting to make your own money.

  It's at this point that you really need to transition from the comfy look of the frat shirts and pajama pants you may have worn in college into a more put-together, casual look. In your twenties you can have fun with fashion. You can overaccessorize—and it will actually work. A pair of shorts with tights, boots, a great sweater, a scarf, a jacket, and a hat will all work in your twenties. You're young and fun and can totally pull it off. Have fun in your twenties figuring out what your fashion style is.

  Trade those pajama pants for a great pair of jeans and your frat shirts for stylish tops. Instead of flip-flops, wear a wedge. Start pulling your look together more.

* In Your Thirties. You have a much better idea of who you are and what your fashion style is. But this is also the time where you might find yourself stuck in a rut. I don't care if you're married or single, or have kids or don't—you're still young! Your fashion should reflect that.

  It's probably time to start steering away from the tattered jeans with holes that worked in your twenties. Switch those for a well-fitting skinny jean and ballet flats or a pair of shorts with a tank and a lightweight jacket.

Honestly, not all rules apply to everyone, but if you're going to wear a white shirt and jeans, pair that with a belt and a cute pair of shoes—and maybe even a scarf. You want your look to be pulled together.

- In Your Forties. I keep hearing forty is the new thirty and I gotta say, I agree! Women in their forties are definitely at their peak. By now, you know who you are and what you like. However, if "who you are and what you like" translates into "I'm afraid of change and I'm going to wear what I always wear," let me give you some pointers to help you get out of your comfort zone.

  Find a pair of straight dark denim jeans. These look great on *every* body type (that's right, you read that correctly). Now find a a solid-colored T-shirt you like. Logos, crazy graphics, and rhinestones are not allowed—just a nice, new cotton T-shirt in a color that looks good on you. Now throw on a ballet flat, wedge, or cute sandal for the summer or a good-quality riding boot in the winter and you're ready to go. And, if it's the winter, trade that T-shirt for a beautiful sweater and a great coat. Throw out any shirts or sweaters in your closet that have started to pill!

  For those of you who work in a casual environment, pair those dark denim jeans with a blazer and heels and you're all set. If you work in a more formal setting, I love a pencil skirt with a crisp button-down shirt—it's chic, elegant, and professional all in one. If skirts aren't your thing, find a good pair of trousers that fit perfectly.

- In Your Fifties, Sixties, and Beyond. Try new things! When I meet women in their fifties and beyond, they are usually pretty set in their ways. I'll hear, "Nope, I can't wear those colors" or "I'll go shopping when I lose ten more pounds" or "I'm too old for that…"

At this point, women are either fashionable or they aren't. They either have a good sense of what looks good on them…or they don't. When they go shopping, they tend to buy more of the same kinds of clothes they already have in their closet. You don't need that same boring cardigan in gray! What you need is that royal blue blouse! Different is good. Go out of your comfort zone a bit.

What *real women* have to say about…

Clothes

"I feel good when the clothes I'm wearing are the right style and fit for me," says Helen.

"I used to be more of a leather boots and jeans kind of girl, but as I've gotten older I've found that I love wearing dresses and skirts," says Nyke. *"It makes me feel very feminine. Dresses are comfortable and classy. You can never go wrong in a dress!"*

"I love jeans, a T-shirt, a fitted jacket, sexy heels, and a hot handbag," says Charlene.

PART III

Live It!

Love yourself first and everything else

falls into line.

—LUCILLE BALL

By now, the real women who have been traveling with you through the pages of this book have learned what they like—and what makes them feel confident and beautiful. In this last, celebratory chapter, everything comes together. And although they enjoy all the pampering from hairdressers, makeup artists, and clothing stylists who helped them glam up for the final photos, they realize they don't need a team of professionals to make them feel and look beautiful. Now, they simply have a few new tools to showcase the best part of themselves—beauty that truly radiates from within. My hope is that after this journey, you, too, will make the same discovery.

A Beautiful Journey

16

I've spent my career turning women into beauty superheroes on magazine covers, on television, and on red carpets. My goal
in this book was to take each of the real women in my life—my family
and friends—on a journey that brought her out of her everyday life,
where she normally *views* beauty images (likes the ones you've seen
in this book) rather than being the subject of them. I wanted these
remarkable women to see themselves as I see them, as *my* beauty
superheroes, and show the world that, although they are regular, *real*
people, just like you and me, their natural, honest beauty is truly "aspirational." I also wanted to present a group of women to the world in
which *you*, beautiful reader, can recognize yourself. It's now time to
come together and celebrate this triumph! Are you with us?!

Getting Ready

It was nearly 5 p.m. at Sarah M.'s house on the final day of the photo shoot for this book. We had spent the last two days—a boot camp of self-recognition and self-triumph—revealing the unique beauty of each of the real women you've seen in these pages and whose voices you've gotten to know.

Sarah's dining room was bustling with activity while we were getting the ladies ready for the final shot. Makeup artists were busy brushing shadow, blush, and powder on the women, highlighting their cheekbones, lining their eyes, swishing on mascara, and putting false eyelashes on a few of them. My team and I were straightening, curling, snipping, and fluffing hair, as well as styling updos, Old Hollywood hair, and French twists. Kayla and her assistant were helping the women pick out the right clothes for them—outfits that fit perfectly and looked oh-so-sexy.

"I feel so special," said Nyke.

Afton said, "I can't believe that's me."

I loved hearing the women say they felt so good. I also loved hearing them talk about themselves, for once, in a positive, genuine, healthy way. I don't always hear that when I'm doing makeovers. They were sharing stories about their accomplishments, their values, how they've looked and felt at different times in their lives, their struggles with hair, weight, and getting older, the men in their lives, their children, their dreams—and how much they learned on our journey together. They were celebrating each other!

The Transformation

When choosing different looks for the ladies, we played up their strengths, personalities, and individual sense of style. I couldn't wait to see the end result, and neither could they. Here's what some of these remarkable women had to say about how they looked and felt.

Lisa

Before stepping out in front of the group, Lisa showed me how she looked in her blue dress. "The blue is just gorgeous," she said. "It's such a great color for me. I never would have thought blue would look so good on me. This dress shows off my curves and makes me look ten pounds thinner!"

Lisa had a subtle, but smoky eye and natural pink lip. Then there was the hair. The night before, I had taken a short, blonde wig and cut it while she was wearing it, giving her a short cropped look that accentuated her neck and jawline but left enough length on top for her to still feel feminine.

I hugged her and took a picture of her myself. I loved how she looked and, more important, how she felt. "Lisa," I said as she stood before me, posing, "I want you to feel the power of your beauty and the power of your body. You are stunning!"

She laughed and started to blush. "Thank you, Ken." I knew she was feeling it!

When she walked into the dining room in the wig, the sexy blue dress, and full makeup, everyone in the room stopped what they were doing to look at her. They lavished her with compliments. They were floored. And so was Lisa. She was literally glowing when she looked in the sprawling mirror in the dining room.

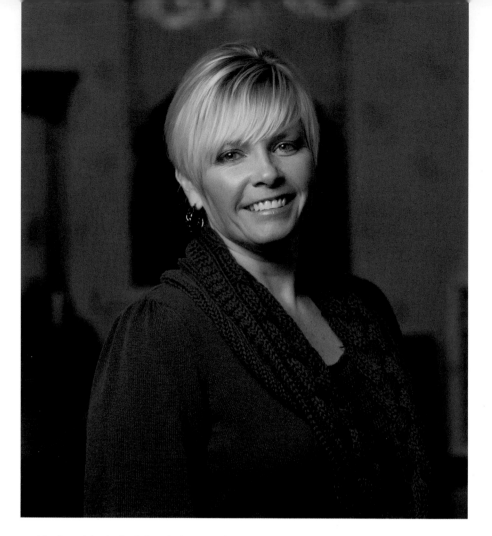

Lisa loved the look of short hair so much that the first thing she did when she returned home was to go to my salon in Michigan and get her hair cut.

Lisa brought me to tears afterward when she took me aside. "Ken, I want to thank you for all this," she said. "I'm going to leave here loving my curves. I'm going to buy a dress like the one I wore today so your brother can take me out. I realize that I look better with bangs or short hair, so I am going to get my hair cut short and go out and get the makeup palette they used on me just now. I just feel great."

Afton

My dear friend Afton has been a force and an amazing influence in my life for many years now. She is so loving and giving. Everything in her life up until now has been about everyone else but her. So this was the perfect time for Afton to come on this journey with us.

Whenever I give her a gift, Afton always says, "This is so perfect. I love that you know me so well." During this journey, she got to know a side of herself that she didn't know she had. Afton's never given herself credit for being beautiful on the outside. She's always covering herself up in layers. But for one of the pictures, we chose a dress that showed off her figure beautifully. She looked great. She came to see that there is also a feminine, curvy woman under there, who doesn't need to hide.

I love that we got Afton out of her comfort zone. She liked the change, too. "For so long, I've done soft and flow-y," Afton said. "So to wear something formfitting is different. I like that this dress fits me so well. I might try going for more formfitting clothes for certain occasions. I'm still going to wear long skirts and flowing shirts and dressy Roman sandals. But I do like the way this kind of dress looks on me." Beauty is about being free to embrace the moment.

Helen

My mom loved the way the fuchsia pink shirt looked on her. The bright pink made her skin glow. We played up her cheeks with a healthy pink glow and added a fuchsia lip stain to accentuate this great color. We played up her eyes with soft neutrals. Helen looked radiant. "I love this color," she said. "The blouse, hair, and makeup make me feel beautiful. It feels pretty great to be me." This reminded me of why I used to love watching my mom do her hair and makeup—she was exuding the inner confidence I always knew she had. We were back to where it all began for me.

Chloe

Seeing how Chloe was beaming made me so happy. Her trademark red lips were the perfect pop of color and paired with a sixties eyeliner on her upper lids, she looked beyond gorgeous with a little hint of edge. Chloe is a confident, beautiful woman. She always has been and always will be. But she had told me she was down on herself a little bit because she had gained a few pounds. Honestly? I didn't even notice. And when she put on those sleek black trousers and that stunning jacket, she looked simply amazing. "I love this!" she said to me. "I feel so great."

Caitlin

Then there was Caitlin, who chose a rose-gold sequined dress that brought out the warmth of her skin tone and was perfect with her Old Hollywood hairstyle. We kept her makeup soft and fresh since her hair was already making a statement. One of the women at the shoot said Caitlin should become an actress because she looked like she belonged on the red carpet.

Here was my niece, breathtaking and red-carpet ready. "I absolutely love this!" she said. Just a few days earlier she was in a T-shirt and jeans, studying at college.

Sarah M.

Sarah looked stunning in a structured dress with dramatic shoulders. The dark gray was subtle in comparison to the strong lines of the dress. Because the collar was so sharply defined, we swept up her rich, vibrant red hair and went with very soft, neutral makeup colors for a chic, sophisticated look. "There is nothing more empowering for a woman than a chic updo and a power dress!" she said.

Nyke

"I feel important, for some reason," Nyke said, loving what she saw. "I have this beautiful, glittery dress on. I love it. I feel like a real woman. I feel really confident. It's great!"

The silver and gold sequin dress Nyke chose went perfectly with her newly lightened auburn locks. "I love how my hair color looks on me," she said. "It makes my skin look rich and glowy." We played up the new, lighter tone of Nyke's hair by going with a red lip color and fresh skin.

Tip

Tip chose a formfitting, deep plum-colored dress that looked beautiful with her luxurious, chestnut locks. She wore her hair down in cascading waves with a soft plum smoky eye and highlighted skin. Tip admitted that she, too, loved all the attention. "I'm usually behind the scenes," she said. "It's nice to be on the other side of things. I love everything we've done today!"

Completing the Journey

Hearing how great each woman felt and how, as a group, they were cheering each other on was everything I hoped this journey together would be. It was so amazing to see the women look at themselves the way they look at women in magazines and in the limelight and realize, "Hey! That's me! I look really good. I can do this!" *You* can look and feel like this too. You just have to recognize how beautiful you already are— the rest is easy!

This was also a journey I had wanted for my mom for a long time. When I picked her up in Michigan to bring her to L.A., she had the winter blues. While we were still in Michigan, I lightened her hair a bit and cut it. Just doing that gave her a lift.

To see my mom, days later, laughing with Caitlin, Lisa, and the other women at the shoot and see her feeling so great about herself made me very happy. When you love someone that much, all you can ask for is for her to love herself as much as you love her. I wanted my mother to see herself the way I see her through my eyes. Later on, when I showed her pictures I had taken of her at the shoot, she joked, "Not bad for a sixty-eight-year-old!" Indeed!

Even Tip, who is already so confident, saw herself in a whole new way. After the shoot, Tip told me how much it meant to her to be included. When I think of true beauty, I always think of Tip. She's never been a model for me in all the years we've worked together. She's never been on a magazine cover or on a red carpet. She's never been celebrated publicly for her beauty, but she is one of the most natural beauties I know.

Still, using her as an example of real beauty today and validating her as a beauty role model took her to a whole different place. She was practically floating around Sarah's house in her glamorous dress, hair, and makeup. She was spinning around and smiling.

The fact that I couldn't get her away from the mirror made me really happy. She loved what she saw. She couldn't get enough of her look. She is naturally confident in her beauty, but knowing that we were sharing her beauty with other people and that we were validating how she already felt about herself was key. It made her soar.

The Final Shot

When everyone was ready, we gathered the ladies in Sarah's formal living room for the final shots of the day. When I walked in and saw how radiant all the women looked, I had to take a deep breath. Each one of them looked so beautiful. Each woman was showcasing herself at her very best, feeling proud of herself and what she looked like. I couldn't ask for more. This is all I had hoped for. Everything had led to this moment.

I had wanted each of these women to realize on her own how beautiful she already is—and then discover how to enhance that beauty—so she could truly feel confident, happy, and comfortable in her own skin. Finally, I wanted each woman to know that she deserves to have her own red carpet moments. It all came full circle for the women—and for me.

Some of the ladies had come to the shoot feeling apprehensive, self-conscious, and unsure of what to expect. But they put their fears aside and tried new things. They learned about new techniques and new looks. When the makeup artists, hair team, and stylists were making them over, they told the women why they used a particular color of shadow, blush, or lip-gloss; why they did their hair a certain way; and

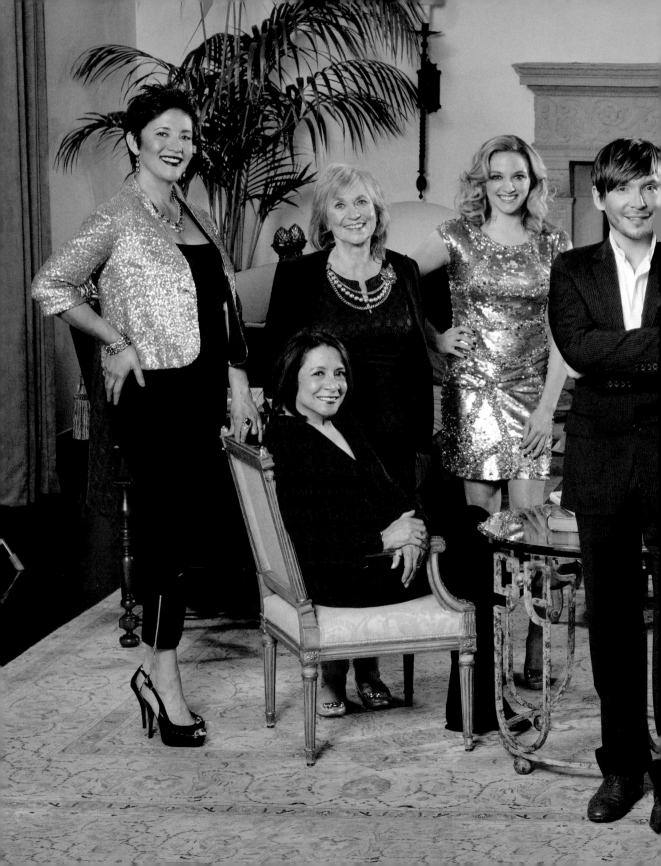

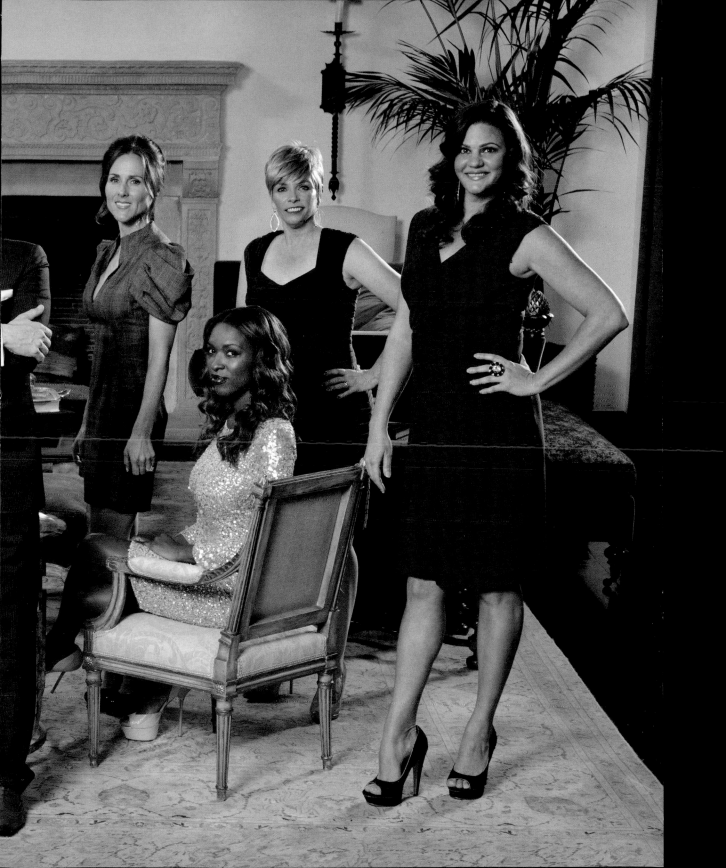

why they suggested those particular outfits. They showed each of the women what works best for her unique beauty.

During this incredible journey, which we took together, I saw so many of the most important women in my life blossom… As a result, they walked away with new self-knowledge, new realizations about themselves. Afton, for example, came to the shoot wanting to wear her own clothes. She was adamant about it. But as time wore on she changed her mind and let the stylist come up with some new options for her. When she saw how beautiful her hair, makeup, and clothes looked, she said to me, almost shyly, "I think I want to start dating again. I think I'm ready to meet a man."

To hear Afton say this made my heart sing. She was in touch with a part of herself that she had been missing for a long time. One of the ladies said that since Afton looked so drop-dead gorgeous that they should go out on the town that night to start looking for a new beau for her—and offered to be Afton's "wing woman." Afton laughed! I think she felt as if she was back in college.

After our friend and world-renowned photographer Richard Maclaren took the final shots of us, I toasted the women with champagne. As we raised our glasses, I said, "Thank you for being here. It means the world to me because I love each and every one of you so much.

"We have taken this incredible journey together and all of you have graduated to a more beautiful you. You've learned so much along the way about yourselves and how to make the most of the unique, natural beauty that all of you possess.

"But guess what? *You don't need me*. You don't need a team of makeup artists and stylists to make you look beautiful. You have everything you need—and you always have. You are beautiful. You always have been. To me, you are what true beauty is today. Cheers, ladies!"

We toasted each other, shed a few happy tears, and hugged each other. Being there with women I love, and seeing them so happy, was one of the most touching moments of my life.

Sisterhood

There was a strong sense of camaraderie and support among the women during our time together. Some of the women knew each other already. Others were meeting for the first time. Over the course of two days, they all bonded. There were lots of laughs, deep discussions, and even a few tears were shed while they shared past experiences and came together over things they had in common. And that is what I want for you, too.

What I loved most is how these women lifted each other up. They oohed and aahed when each of them came into the dining room sporting a particularly daring, gorgeous look. They hugged each other. They jokingly called each other "Hot mama" and "Sexy thing." They were there for each other in spirit. I would like all women to treat each other like that. So many women are competing over who looks better. Pitting women against each other is unproductive. Life's too short. Live your life. Lift each other up. Support each other. Let the competitiveness go. Accept yourself and other women for who they are. In order to see yourself as beautiful, you need to see others as beautiful.

Most of all, take what you learn about accepting yourself and being the best you can be—and share it with other women to help them recognize their own unique, natural beauty. When you are confident enough in your own beauty, then you can compliment others and really mean it. When you find beauty in other people, you find it in yourself.

Your Own Beautiful Journey

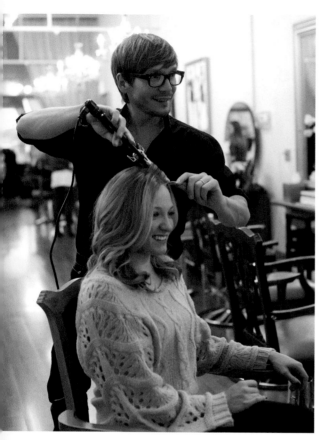

Finishing the toast and saying our goodbyes was the end of a beautiful journey the ladies and I took together. But for you, my friend? Your journey is only just beginning. I hope you use this book as a springboard to a happier, healthier you. I hope you finally see just how special you are and how much you have to offer. It all starts with loving yourself first. All of you. Acknowledge and love yourself today because when tomorrow comes, you may regret that you didn't enjoy what you already have. Be in the present. Celebrate yourself now!

And by the way, I want to let you know that like the real women in my life, you don't need me, either. You don't need teams of stylists to make you beautiful. You have everything you need to be the best you possible. Cheers, my friend. You are beautiful—*just as you've always been.*

Giving Back

One of the things that I find most beautiful and that fills my heart is helping others, whether volunteering time with a charity or taking a moment to share some caring words with someone else. I've always believed that we need to be there for each other and lift each other up when we can. My feeling is that you cannot truly give to yourself unless you give of yourself. Giving to others gives me purpose and value as a human being. It is healing for me and helps me appreciate all the blessings I have in my life and all those who have helped me. Without the help of many others, I would not be living my dreams today. I am humbled and beyond grateful.

I hope to make a difference, whether as a voice of realistic, nonjudgmental beauty or as an ambassador for philanthropy. Since I was a child, I wanted to stand up for children who didn't have a voice or couldn't stand up for themselves. My father always taught me to stand up for myself and my mother taught me that I mattered. Now, because of the success I've had with my career, I will use my voice to be heard.

My Inspiration

When my nephew Ryan was born in 1988, he changed my life. Ryan was a gift from God for my family and me. He was a little angel; he was all love. Ryan loved us unconditionally and taught us to love unconditionally. What made Ryan even more unique was that he was born different, with several birth defects. This may have made him physically "different" from you and me, but he was perfectly Ryan. He was—and still is—a constant reminder of what is truly beautiful in life. Because of Ryan, I find "unique" to be more beautiful than "normal."

It was definitely no mistake that God intended Ryan to be with my brother, Jon, and his wife, Lisa, whom you've gotten to know in these pages. God knew Jon and Lisa would love, honor, nurture, and cherish Ryan with the dignity and respect he deserved. Ryan was their first child and they were so proud. They celebrated every moment with him while he was here on earth and took him everywhere. They didn't try to hide Ryan or shield the world from him. Here was a child that others may not have seen as "normal," but Jon and Lisa gave him a life that I think was better than normal. Jon, Lisa, and Ryan taught me one of the greatest lessons I've ever learned—that no matter what, you are you, the way God intended you to be, and there is no reason to hide and every reason to live and appreciate life. Jon and Lisa have three other children—Caitlin, whom you've also met here; Chloe, who's twelve and, I always say, my twin; and Ethan, who's nineteen and also looks just like me, though he's a lot taller—but no one ever forgets about Ryan, ever.

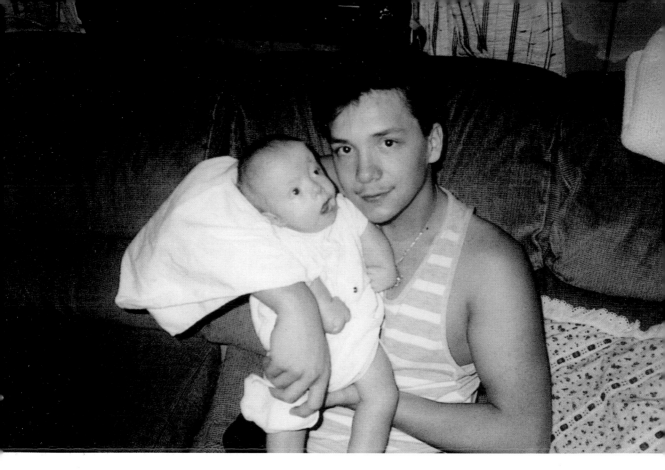

Ryan and me

Imperfectly Perfect

Ryan was born with a chromosomal disorder called trisomy 18. He had four fingers, which were webbed, and no thumbs. My brother Jon— who always finds the positive in everything and who loved his boy so much—would always say to Ryan, "Give me a high four!" Ryan also had no wrists; his ears were not fully formed, and he was hearing impaired; he had a cleft lip and a high arched palate and was fed through a tube in his stomach; he had hydrocephalus and a hole in his heart, which would later cause his heart to stop and Ryan to leave us. He was imperfectly perfect, the way God had intended him to be, and I loved him more than anything. It was hard not to. Ryan was so full of life and love. He was all smiles, always happy. You couldn't see him or hold him without smiling yourself. And believe me, we held him all the time. We loved making Ryan laugh. We cuddled him nonstop. Ryan lit up when we danced and played with him. I used to sing and hum to Ryan with his head on my shoulder and my cheek against his—I think he liked the vibration of the humming.

My Greatest Role Model

When Ryan was born, I had no idea that a child who would live such a short time would become one of my greatest teachers. Ryan was here with us for only fifteen months, but he lived beyond everyone's expectations. He was always a reminder of what you could do, not what you couldn't do. He empowered many of us—including me—to do whatever we want in life because he did things he was never expected to do. We were told, for example, that he would live only three months, yet he made it to fifteen months. He was never supposed to make it to that first Christmas, yet he made it to two. We even got to celebrate his first tooth.

These things might seem inconsequential, but they were huge accomplishments that made me realize that I could do anything I want to do—especially helping others—as long as it comes from a place of love, passion, purpose, and goodness.

Ryan reminded all of us who knew him to love life, cherish every moment, and celebrate every accomplishment, no matter how large or small. For many people today, an achievement has to be gigantic—supersized—for it to matter. But everything Ryan did was special, from his sweet smile to the littlest wave of his hand. He is still a constant reminder to keep things in perspective and to celebrate yourself, every day.

Honoring Ryan

When Ryan died, Jon and Lisa called us over to the house to say goodbye. We got to hold him one last time. I thought for sure that if I hugged him enough, I could love him back to life and make him open his eyes.

Saying goodbye to Ryan was one of the hardest things I've ever done. I was only seventeen and didn't understand why this had happened. I missed Ryan more than anything. I still do. Even writing this is difficult for me. I have a tattoo of an angel—Ryan—on my arm. The angel tattoo was picked out by Ryan's sister Caitlin and his brother Ethan. Ryan is always with me. I believe he's had a hand in everything good that has ever happened to me.

Ryan's passing only confirmed that I wanted to spend my life helping children. SOFT, the Support Organization for Trisomy, is an amazing organization that helped and informed Jon, Lisa, and our whole family about trisomy. I want to say thank you, SOFT, on behalf of my family and me, and especially Ryan.

From the moment Ryan died, I promised myself that I would spend the rest of my life honoring him and that I would never let his life go unrecognized. He had done so much for so many people in his own way. I knew that my job was to be a messenger for what he taught all of us who were blessed to know him—to recognize the good in life, to appreciate every moment, to be grateful for what you have and for the people in your life, to strive to be the best you can be, and to help others, especially children. I feel that I've been able to help other children along the way because of Ryan, who, even as an angel in heaven, is still helping thousands of people—especially children.

Give Wherever You Can

Over the years, I've worked with many amazing charities, such as Rally for Kids With Cancer, the Rainbow Connection, Padres Contra El Cancer, and the Greater Los Angeles Agency on Deafness, among others. For years, I've donated wigs to cancer patients who need them.

One of the most inspiring and courageous people I've met in my life is twenty-two-year-old Rachel Nasuti. She has epidermolysis bullosa, a disorder caused by a genetic mutation that causes the skin (or other organs) to blister. Even a minor scratch or nick can cause excruciating pain and bleeding—making everyday tasks like eating, drinking, and holding things incredibly challenging. Severe scarring can cause deformities in the hands and feet, thus the need to wear bandages at all times to prevent injury and infection. An estimated 100,000 Americans suffer from EB, according to the Epidermolysis Bullosa Medical Research Foundation (EBMRF). Many of those affected are children. Kids with this disorder are known as "butterfly children" since their skin is as fragile as a butterfly's wings.

Like Ryan, Rachel (who was thirteen when we met) has become a teacher and a role model for me because she doesn't define herself by EB. So many of us focus on what we can't do or can't be. Rachel always looks at the positive side of things. She doesn't let anything stop her. EB hasn't kept her from embracing life and living it to the fullest.

I had a chance to recognize Rachel and EB when Oprah Winfrey invited me to *Give Big* in January 2006. I decided to "give big" to EB and partnered with a great team, including Andrea Pett-Joseph and her husband Paul Joseph—who founded EBMRF because their son Brandon has EB—and my friend Eva Longoria, who graciously allowed us to hold a fund-raiser at her restaurant, Beso.

Jennifer Aniston, Kate Beckinsale, Orlando Bloom, Jessica and Ashlee Simpson, Holly Robinson-Peete, Jason Bateman, Courteney Cox, and David Arquette, among others, came to the event to support the cause. Nate Burkus, who hosted *Oprah's Big Give*, also came out in support.

We raised an unbelievable $2.2 million for EB. An anonymous donor pledged $1 million, and Stiefel Laboratories, a manufacturer of products for the care and treatment of skin diseases, matched that pledge with another $1 million donation. We also held a live auction, with eBay. We auctioned items from Bette Midler, The Eagles, Christina Aguilera, David and Victoria Beckham, Jessica and Ashlee Simpson, Celine Dion, Satya jewelry, and many others.

Follow Your Heart

I'm also proud to be an ambassador for Operation Smile (OS), whose doctors travel the world, fixing major facial deformities, usually cleft lips and palates, for free. Seeing how happy the people are after their surgeries is one of the most rewarding things I have ever experienced.

In 2004, I traveled to Honduras for an OS mission. Caitlin, who was only thirteen, came with me. She told me she wanted to go for Ryan. Caitlin brought small plastic sandwich bags filled with jacks, balls, and other small toys to give to the children. Our main role was to bring ease to the families, play with and comfort the children, and show them to and from their appointments and screenings to see if they were healthy enough for surgery. Caitlin and I spent hours playing, laughing, and bonding with all the kids. We fell in love especially with a young girl named Dianna. She was so happy, full of life, and had no idea that she didn't look like everyone else. What a contrast with Los Angeles, where if someone has a bad hair day it becomes breaking news.

As an ambassador for Operation Smile I was invited to scrub in on the surgeries (outside of the U.S.), which opened my eyes to the miracles that the amazing Operation Smile team performs. Caitlin had the opportunity to scrub in, too, and at thirteen years old became the youngest person at the time to attend a facial cranial surgery. She did it for Ryan and Dianna. It was healing for her and for me. As a result, Caitlin has decided to go to college and study nursing.

I have been working with Operation Smile since 2002. In 2005, OS gave me its Smile of Hope Award at a benefit back home in Michigan. I accepted the award on behalf of Ryan and gave it to his parents, Jon and Lisa, who were there that evening. It was a dream come true to honor my nephew in our hometown and to celebrate his parents—a moment I will never forget.

Again, I begged and borrowed auction items to raise money for Operation Smile, and once again, generous hearts rallied. Oprah and *The Oprah Winfrey Show* donated tickets to the show, which we auctioned for $10,000, and Celine Dion gave tickets to her show, which also went for $10,000. It was a successful night. The event, in part, sponsored an OS mission to Kenya and allowed Operation Smile to sponsor a young Kenyan girl, named Mercy, at the University of Michigan Health System. Her case was rather severe and she could not be operated on at the OS site in Kenya. I met Mercy at the event and spent time with her in Michigan and, later, in Kenya. Mercy was also a small warrior, carrying a large burden.

I introduced Jessica Simpson to Operation Smile in 2003. She took on the role of International Youth Ambassador. She was passionate about OS and became one of its most vocal and active supporters. Jessica's involvement in Operation Smile gained international interest, and in March 2006, we had the great honor of traveling to Washington, DC, with a delegation from OS, including its founder, Dr. William Magee, to meet with members of Congress and lobby for the charity.

This was a moment when I had to take pause. Jessica and I wouldn't have been there on Capitol Hill if it weren't for Ryan. I had tried to honor my nephew my whole life. Here I was, before Congress, lobbying for OS in Ryan's name. His life would help other children with cleft lips and palates. I think he would have been proud to know that his life had a greater purpose than just living for fifteen months.

I'm so grateful to Operation Smile for allowing me to help it do its life-changing work. I am also grateful to Jessica for lending her name and her heart to Operation Smile, for me, for Ryan, and for thousands of children around the world.

How You Can Help—in Big Ways and Small

Years ago, I decided that one of my life's purposes was to give back to others. I made a vow that I would do whatever I could—I wasn't going to wait until I had millions of dollars to donate and I would never say no. I would give what I could, no matter how big or small.

Give what you have to give; it can be money, but it doesn't have to be. You can give your time, your energy, your passion; a kind and helping hand goes a long way. I often donate services at my salons for auctions to raise money. We have a responsibility as human beings on this earth to help each other—to look into the eyes of people in need and give them the honor and respect they deserve, that we all deserve.

We all have gifts to share. There's nothing better in life than feeling that you have a purpose that's greater than just yourself. Giving is contagious. The moment you start doing something for others, you find that the universe gives back to you. We all need help sometime!

You don't have to start your own global charity. You can lend a hand in your own backyard. There are so many things you can do. If you bought a little too much of something, give it to a neighbor who might need it. Give someone a much-needed smile or hug or some words of encouragement. You can donate used coats, clothes, and other things you don't need to those who do. You can help feed someone by bringing them food along with plates and plastic silverware wrapped in napkins, which gives them dignity as well as nourishment.

So many people go through life selfishly rather than selflessly. When you find a greater purpose in life beyond yourself, a balance between you and the universe, you really begin to feel happy and experience a true sense of worth. I think true happiness comes when you realize, "Wow. I'm a part of something greater than myself." People who are truly happy are serving a greater purpose. That is beautiful.

ACKNOWLEDGMENTS

Thank you to everyone who encouraged me along the way, and who believed in me, before I had the courage to believe in myself.

My love and sincerest gratitude to:

My Mom Helen, for all your love and always believing in and encouraging me—Mommy and I are one! My Dad Gary for always accepting me, loving me for me, and teaching me to work around the clock. My brothers Chris and Jon for always letting me tag along and be the coolest one in the bunch! Martin, this book would not have been possible without you. More than life itself!

The amazing women of this book, who inspired me with their truth: Tip, Audrey, Caitlin, Charlene, Lisa, Sarah M, Chloe, Afton, Nyke, Lesli, Blair, and Sarah L! My dear friend Claudia who doesn't appear in this book but is definitely a big part of it! I adore you. Jan Miller, Nena Madonia, and Dupre Miller & Associates for believing I had something to say.

Jennifer Williams, Michael Fragnito, Elizabeth Mihaltse, and everyone at Sterling Publishing and Buoy Point Media for fulfilling this dream.

K.C. Baker for your tireless dedication! Gary Magness and Sarah Siegel Magness for allowing me to photograph at your lovely home, Casa Mango. Richard Mclaren, for your beautiful pictures. Ken Paves Salon team for all your hard work! Stila cosmetics for making my ladies look so pretty! Kayla Mcgee for your style!

This is not my book it is ours. You Are Beautiful!

Index

INDEX